The Prevention of Food Poisoning

Fourth Edition

Jill Trickett

First published in 1978 by:
Stanley Thornes (Publishers) Ltd
Second edition 1986
Third edition 1992

Fourth edition published in 2001 by:
Nelson Thornes Ltd
Delta Place
27 Bath Road
CHELTENHAM
GL53 7TH
United Kingdom

01 02 03 04 05 / 10 9 8 7 6 5 4 3

A catalogue record for this book is available from the British Library

ISBN 0 7487 5893 3

Illustrations by Angela Lumley
Page make-up by Columns Design Ltd

Printed and bound in Great Britain by T.J. International

Contents

Preface to the fourth edition

My aim in writing this book is quite simply to provide an introduction to the subject of food poisoning. The fact that the number of outbreaks of food poisoning is increasing each year, despite apparently higher living standards and high standards of personal hygiene, suggests that many people working in the food industry and also many who prepare food at home have incomplete knowledge of the causes and prevention of food poisoning.

The book seeks to offer an interesting and logical approach to the basic principles of preventing food poisoning and food-borne diseases. No previous knowledge of the subject is required but for anyone already acquainted with the basic ideas, the provision of subheadings and cross-references should make it possible to refer to any particular subject area.

This new edition includes a chapter on travel and food-related illnesses, a subject that is becoming more important as the number of people travelling abroad for business and for holidays increases. There is also a new chapter about food hazard analysis, the food industry's approach to reducing food-poisoning outbreaks.

The book covers the syllabuses of The Royal Institute of Public Health and Hygiene Certificate in Food Hygiene and Safety and The Chartered Institute of Environmental Health Level 2 Intermediate Food Hygiene examination. It provides a good groundwork for more advanced examinations but remains a readable text for those who are not taking examinations but merely wish to understand the principles of the prevention of food poisoning.

J. Trickett   *Summer 2001*

Acknowledgements

The author would like to thank:

Mr R R Charnock of The College, Swindon, who first suggested that I should write this book; to him and Mrs B D Martin, who read the manuscript, making a number of suggestions.

Ian Greaves (I.G.I. Consultants) and John Frater (Chief Executive of the Royal Environmental Health Institute of Scotland) for advice on the manuscript of the fourth edition and to John Frater for contributing the material on food hygiene legislation in Scotland in Chapter 22.

The author and publishers would like to thank the following people and organisations for permission to reproduce the following material:

C & C Catering Equipment Ltd for the signs on pages 108, 109 and 114; The Department of Health for posters on pages 73, 149 and 150; Digital Stock for the photo on page 4; Ian Greaves International for photos on pages 95 and 135; Jan Hobot/Wellcome Photo Library for the photo on page 40; Lockhart Catering Equipment for photos on pages 90, 105 and 113; The Public Health Legislation Service Communicable Disease Surveillance Centre for information on pages 51, 54, 80 and 81; Rentokil Initial for photos on pages 117, 119, 120, 121 and 122; and The Wellcome Photo Library for photos on pages 29, 35 and 46.

Every effort has been made to contact copyright holders, and we apologise if any have been overlooked.

1 WHAT IS FOOD POISONING?

Everybody expects to be provided with food which is safe to eat but unfortunately this does not always happen and the number of cases of food poisoning and food-borne disease increases most years. If this trend is to be reversed it is important that people working in the food industry and those who prepare food at home should make sure that they are fully aware of the best methods of handling and preparing food.

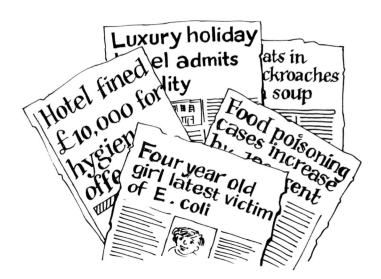

Most cases of food poisoning are caused by eating food contaminated with large numbers of pathogenic (harmful) bacteria but food poisoning can also be caused by viruses, chemicals, poisonous plants and fish.

The symptoms of food poisoning are usually vomiting, diarrhoea and abdominal pains. Vomiting and diarrhoea are the body's method of disposing of harmful substances from the digestive tract, thus preventing them from getting into the bloodstream.

How common is food poisoning?

The number of reported cases of food poisoning has almost doubled in the last ten years despite apparently higher standards of hygiene and increased awareness of the causes of food poisoning. It is estimated that there are at least ten times and possibly as many as 100 times as many cases which are not reported and are therefore not included in these figures.

There are a number of reasons for this increase.

1　Intensive rearing of farm animals such as chickens and pigs. Because the animals are so crowded, bacteria spread from one to another. The meat we buy is therefore contaminated with pathogenic bacteria.

2　The practice of eating out is becoming far more popular and the majority of the working population is eating at least one meal a day in a restaurant, pub or canteen or buying a sandwich from a shop. If a mistake is made in food preparation in one of these catering establishments a large number of people will be affected, whereas a similar incident in the home will affect only a small number of people.

Starters

Garlic ciabatta roll with spicy pepper salsa	£2.95
Homemade soup	£3.45
Lamb samosas with peanut chilli dressing	£3.95
Potato skins with garlic mayonnaise	£3.95

Main courses

Warm chicken salad with a sweet chilli, garlic and mint sauce	£6.25
Caesar salad with chargrilled salmon	£7.25
Pasta Romano with roasted tomato, basil and pine nut sauce	£7.65
Cured pork hotpot in apricot, pepper and mustard sauce	£9.95
Seafood platter	£9.95
Marinated duck with flour tortillas, guacamole and salsa	£10.95
Grilled sirloin steak with fries, coleslaw and corn salsa	£11.95

Desserts

Warm toffee cheesecake	£4.35
Dark and white chocolate mousse	£3.95
Marinated exotic fruit with a vanilla sauce	£3.95
Chocolate mud pie	£4.35

3   Restaurants, canteens, etc. produce a much more varied range of dishes than used to be the case. With this degree of choice, instead of food being served hot immediately after it is cooked, there is a tendency to keep foods warm until a customer requests a particular dish.

4   There has been a rapid growth in the number of shops selling take-away meals. The food is frequently cooked in advance and then reheated on purchase. If it is not cooled quickly and stored in a refrigerator between cooking and reheating there will be plenty of opportunity for bacterial growth.

DANSAK DISHES
A sweet & sour curry cooked with lintils & pineapples

97.	Chicken	3.50	98.	Keema	3.50
99.	Lamb or Beef	3.50	100.	Vegetable	3.20
101.	Prawn	3.50	102.	Mushroom	2.95
101.	Chicken Tikka	3.95	104.	King Prawn	4.50
105.	Lamb Tikka	3.95	106.	Special Mix	4.50

PATHIA DISHES
A sour & hot taste using fresh tomatoes, onions, garlic and black pepper

138.	Chicken Tikka	3.95	139.	Chicken	3.50
140.	Lamb	3.50	141.	Beef	3.95
142.	Prawn	3.50	143.	King Prawn	4.50

ENGLISH DISHES
Served with green salad, peas & chips

144.	Fried Scampi	3.80	145.	Fried chicken	3.80
146.	Chicken Omelette	3.50	147.	Prawn Omelette	3.50
148.	Mushroom Omelette	3.50			

MEDIUM CURRY DISHES
Cooked with fresh spices

149.	Chicken Tikka	3.65	150.	Lamb	3.25
151.	Lamb Tikka	3.65	152.	Chicken	3.25
153.	Keema	2.80	154.	Prawn	3.25
155.	Meat	3.50	156.	King Prawn	4.00
157.	Vegetable	3.20	158.	Special Mix	3.95

MADRAS DISHES
Hot curry with spices

159.	Chicken Tikka	3.95	160.	Lamb	3.50
161.	Lamb Tikka	3.95	162.	Chicken	3.50
163.	Keema	3.20	164.	Prawn	3.25
165.	Meat	3.50	166.	King Prawn	4.50
167.	Vegetable	3.20	168.	Special Mix	4.50

5   Large-scale factory production of foods has led to an increase in food poisoning. Although factory processes are normally very carefully controlled, a slight error at some stage in production could lead to thousands of contaminated prepacked foods which may be distributed throughout the country.

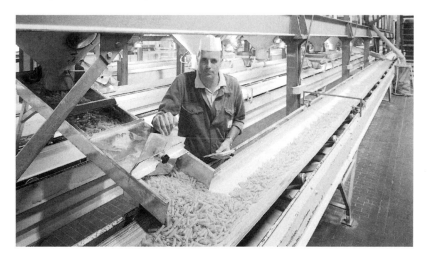

6   People tend to shop for food weekly rather than daily, resulting in a greater chance of bacterial growth in the food after purchase unless it is stored correctly. Meals are sometimes cooked ahead of requirements and reheated when needed which increases the chance for bacterial growth.

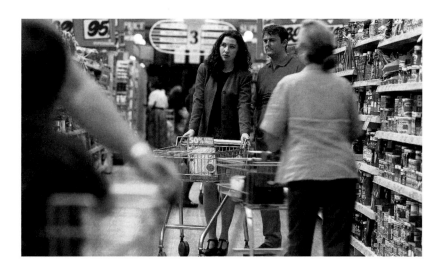

7   The majority of outbreaks of food poisoning occur during the summer months. In the summer, there is an increased tendency to pack foods, for picnics and for journeys to holiday resorts. These are often kept at warm temperatures for several hours before they are eaten. Insulated bags and ice boxes should be used to keep food cool if it will not be eaten for several hours after removal from the refrigerator. Inadequate cooking of meat on a barbecue is a common cause of food poisoning. In addition, eating outside attracts flies, which present a hygiene problem.

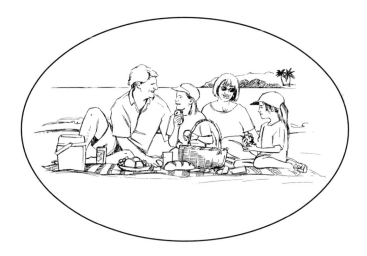

8   Untrained staff are often employed during the summer months to cope with the increased demand for restaurant meals. All staff should be taught the basic principles of food hygiene and should be carefully supervised in their first few weeks' work.

Summary

- ❑ Most cases of food poisoning are caused by bacteria.
- ❑ The symptoms of food poisoning are usually vomiting, diarrhoea and abdominal pains.

❏ The number of cases of food poisoning is increasing due to:
  (a) intensive rearing of farm animals
  (b) an increased tendency to eat out
  (c) a much more varied menu
  (d) an increasing number of shops selling take-away meals
  (e) large-scale factory production of food
  (f) an increased tendency to shop and cook several days in advance of eating.

❏ The majority of outbreaks of food poisoning occur in the summer months.

❏ It is very important for all food handlers to be trained in food hygiene.

2 MICROBIOLOGY

Microbiology is the study of micro-organisms. *Micro-organism* is a general term for a small living creature which cannot be seen without using a microscope. Micro-organisms are found everywhere: in food, water, soil, air and on and in human and animal bodies. Many micro-organisms are completely harmless to humans and can be present in food without having any undesirable effect. Some even perform useful functions.

The micro-organisms frequently found in food fall into four main categories:
❑ bacteria
❑ yeasts
❑ moulds
❑ viruses.

Bacteria

It is useful to divide the bacteria commonly found in food into three groups:
❑ pathogens
❑ spoilage bacteria
❑ useful bacteria.

Pathogens

Only a few of the thousands of different types of bacteria cause illness. Those which do are known as *pathogens*. The presence of pathogens in food causes either food poisoning or a food-borne disease (see p. 27).

Food can contain large numbers of pathogenic bacteria and yet look, smell and taste perfectly wholesome. In order to prevent bacterial food poisoning it is important to understand the factors which favour the growth of these pathogens and the way in which they are spread to food (see p. 10).

Spoilage bacteria

Certain bacteria are capable of spoiling food without make it poisonous. The change in odour, taste and appearance of pasteurised milk on keeping is due to acids produced by bacteria as they grow in the milk. Meat and fish start to smell and become slimy due to the waste products of the bacteria that are growing on them. Spoilage bacteria are not usually pathogenic. However, if food has been kept in conditions which allow the multiplication of spoilage bacteria, any food-poisoning bacteria which are also present are likely to have had a chance to multiply.

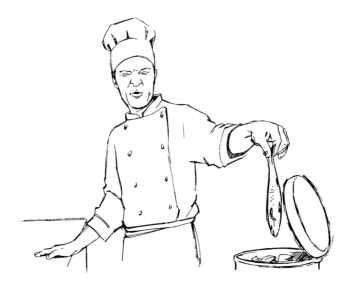

Useful bacteria

Many bacteria perform useful functions and are essential for certain processes, for example:
❑　the manufacture of cheese and yoghurt
❑　the production of some antibiotics and some vitamins
❑　the production of manure from decaying vegetable matter.

Yeasts

Yeasts do not cause food poisoning but some types are capable of causing food spoilage. They usually spoil acid foods with a high sugar content, e.g.

fruit juices, yoghurts, wines. One type of yeast has great commercial importance because it is used for the production of bread and alcohol (beer, wine and cider).

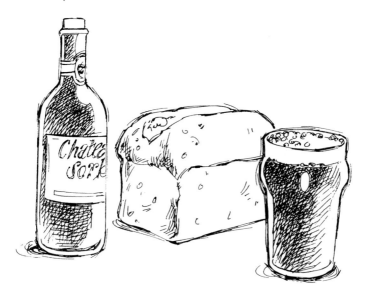

Moulds

Moulds do not normally cause food poisoning although some of them can produce *mycotoxins* (poisonous substances). Moulds present in grain or nuts which are stored in damp conditions produce mycotoxins which may cause cancer. Food is frequently spoiled by moulds, particularly fairly dry or acid food. Black or blue-green moulds are a familiar sight on bread and citrus fruits. Some moulds are used in the production of antibiotics and blue cheeses.

Viruses

These are much smaller than bacteria and can only be seen with an electron microscope. They only multiply in living tissue and will not multiply in food. If certain viruses enter the body they may cause food poisoning with the typical symptoms of vomiting and diarrhoea (see p. 59).

Characteristics of bacteria

Bacteria are so small that they can be seen only through a microscope. Approximately one million bacteria clumped together would cover a pin-head. A bacterium has a very simple structure consisting of one cell only whereas the human body (or that of any animal or insect) is made up of countless numbers of different cells.

There are many different types of bacteria and they vary in shape and size but the ones found in food are usually spherical (*cocci*) or rod-shaped (*bacilli*).

COCCUS
A spherical or near
spherical cell, e.g. staphylococcus

BACILLUS
A rod-shaped cell, longer
than it is broad, e.g. salmonella

Bacteria are present almost everywhere: in the air, on our skin and hair, in our noses and mouths, in our intestinal tracts, in our food, on kitchen equipment, in garden soil and in water. Some are mobile and can swim around in liquids but most cannot move by themselves. These are only transferred by direct contact.

Growth and multiplication

If bacteria are supplied with food, water and a warm temperature, they will grow and reproduce by a process known as *binary fission*. The bacterial cell grows to a maximum size by absorbing simple substances from its environment and then splits into two new identical cells. In optimum conditions (the very best conditions) for growth bacteria will divide into two approximately every 20 minutes.

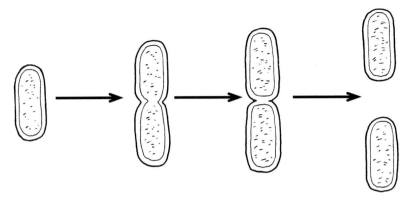

Bacteria reproduce by a process known as binary fission

One bacterium will therefore produce two bacteria after 20 minutes. These two bacteria will then both grow and divide into two after a further 20 minutes, making a total of four bacteria after 40 minutes. After 60 minutes there will be eight bacteria and after five or six hours there will be thousands of bacteria.

Study the following table to see how quickly the number of bacteria in food can increase. Can you fill in the spaces?

	20 min	40 min	60 min
0 hours	2	4	8
1 hour	16	32	64
2 hours	128	256	
3 hours	1024	2048	4096
4 hours		16 384	
5 hours	65 536		262 144

After six hours in optimum conditions it is possible for one bacterium to become 262 144 bacteria. These bacteria will continue to grow at the same rate until food or an essential growth factor is no longer available or until the presence of poisonous waste products inhibits their growth.

Bacterial spores

When bacteria are growing and multiplying we say they are in the *vegetative state*. In this state they are fairly easily destroyed by heat or chemicals. Some bacteria, but not all, can exist in another form – the *spore* form. A spore is a rounded body which forms inside the bacterial cell when conditions become unfavourable for growth or multiplication. The rest of the cell then gradually disintegrates, leaving only the spore. These spores can resist very high temperatures and high concentrations of chemicals that would kill bacteria in the vegetative state. They can survive at least four hours in boiling water and so they are not destroyed by normal cooking methods. Spores are also formed when there is insufficient moisture present. They can survive for years without food or water but when conditions become favourable the spores return to the vegetative state and continue to grow and multiply.

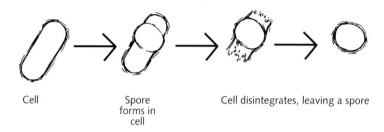

Cell   Spore   Cell disintegrates, leaving a spore
forms in
cell

Bacterial toxins

Some bacteria produce *toxins* (poisonous substances) whilst they are growing and multiplying in food. Any toxin which affects the intestinal tract is called an *enterotoxin*. Enterotoxins are divided into exotoxins and endotoxins.

❏ *Exotoxins* are produced by bacteria whilst they are living and growing in food. They are released from the bacterial cell and are sometimes more heat resistant than the cell itself. Food poisoning can be caused by food containing bacterial exotoxins although there are no live bacteria present. The incubation period is short because the exotoxin causes vomiting soon after the food is eaten. The main symptom is vomiting, but this may be followed by diarrhoea and abdominal pains (see Staphylococcus food poisoning, p. 35).

❏ *Endotoxins* form part of the bacterial cell and are released on the death of the bacterial cell during digestion of the contaminated food. The incubation period is longer than with food poisoning caused by exotoxins and the main sympton is diarrhoea. See *Clostridium perfringens* food poisoning (p. 40).

Aerobes and anaerobes

Bacteria differ from one another in their requirements for oxygen. Some of them require the presence of air to grow and multiply and these are called *aerobes* (see *Bacillus cereus*, p. 46).

Some will grow and multiply faster in the absence of oxygen. These are called *anaerobes* (see *Clostridium perfringens*, p. 40). Some will not multiply at all in the presence of oxygen and these are called *obligate anaerobes* (see *Clostridium botulinum*, p. 57).

Some can multiply equally well in the presence or absence of oxygen and these are called *facultative anaerobes* (see Salmonella, p. 29).

Summary

- ❏ Bacteria, yeasts, moulds and viruses are all micro-organisms which are frequently present in food.

- ❏ In optimum conditions for growth, bacterial cells will divide into two new cells approximately every 20 minutes.

- ❏ Some bacteria form spores when conditions are not suitable for multiplication.

- ❏ Some bacteria produce enterotoxins.

- ❏ Bacteria differ in their requirement for air.

3 THE GROWTH REQUIREMENTS OF FOOD-POISONING BACTERIA

In order to grow and multiply all bacteria require four things: warmth, food, moisture and time.

Warmth

Optimum temperature

The bacteria which cause food poisoning prefer to live at the temperature of the human body (37°C) and it is at this temperature that they will grow and multiply at the fastest rate. They will, however, multiply throughout the temperature range 5–63°C, which is called the *DANGER ZONE*.

High temperatures

As the temperature increases from 37°C to 63°C the rate of growth slows down and at temperatures above 63°C bacteria will gradually be killed. The length of time and the temperature required to kill them will depend on the type of bacteria and the food involved. They are normally killed in 1–2 minutes in boiling water, unless they are able to form spores, in which case they may survive up to 4–5 hours in boiling water.

Low temperatures

If the temperature of the food is decreased from 37°C to 5°C the bacteria will continue to multiply but the rate of multiplication will slow down as the temperature decreases. Bacteria are not killed by low temperatures but they are dormant. This means that they stay alive but stop growing and multiplying. Most food-poisoning bacteria will not grow at the temperature of the domestic refrigerator (1–4°C) but some spoilage bacteria are able to grow and multiply slowly. When the foods are removed from the refrigerator, the rate of bacterial growth increases, as the temperature increases.

Frozen food

Bacteria can remain dormant even in frozen food but as soon as the food is thawed they will start to grow and multiply again.

Room temperatures

The average room temperature is 20°C but in the summer, the temperature in a badly ventilated kitchen can reach 30°C, at which bacteria can multiply

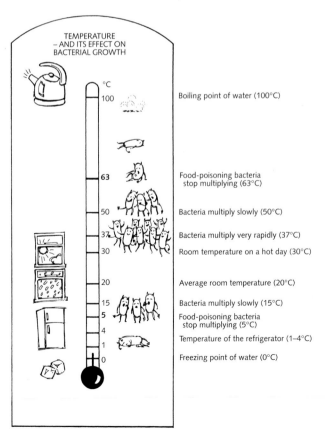

TEMPERATURE
– AND ITS EFFECT ON
BACTERIAL GROWTH

°C

100 — Boiling point of water (100°C)

63 — Food-poisoning bacteria stop multiplying (63°C)

50 — Bacteria multiply slowly (50°C)

37 — Bacteria multiply very rapidly (37°C)

30 — Room temperature on a hot day (30°C)

20 — Average room temperature (20°C)

15 — Bacteria multiply slowly (15°C)

5 — Food-poisoning bacteria stop multiplying (5°C)

4
1 — Temperature of the refrigerator (1–4°C)

0 — Freezing point of water (0°C)

very rapidly. For this reason foods should not be allowed to stand for any length of time in a kitchen. Any preparation should be done as quickly as possible and then the food should be stored in a refrigerator until it is ready to be served.

Food

Like all living things bacteria need food. They will live and multiply in many foodstuffs, particularly those which are high in protein and moisture and have a near-neutral pH (see p. 124). The foods that most frequently cause food poisoning are called *high-risk foods*.

1　Meats, poultry and meat products (meat pies and pasties, sausages).

2　Stocks, gravies, stews and sauces.

3　Milk, cream and egg products (custards, trifles).

The following foods do not normally cause food poisoning and are called *low-risk foods*.

1　Acid foods (pickles, citrus fruits).

2　Foods with a high concentration of salt (salted meats, anchovies, olives).

3　Foods with a high concentration of sugar (jams, syrups).

4　Fatty foods (butter, cooking oil).

5　Dry foods (biscuits, flour).

Although bacteria thrive on foods enjoyed by humans, a crumb lodged in a crack on a table or a smear of blood on an unwashed chopping board is sufficient food for thousands of bacteria.

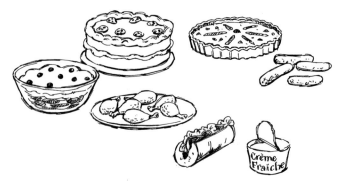

Some of the foods which support bacterial growth

Moisture

Like all living things bacteria require moisture for growth. Most foods contain sufficient water for bacterial growth but dehydrated products such as milk powder, dried soup powder and dried egg powder will not allow the growth of bacteria. In dried products bacteria survive but remain dormant until the powders are reconstituted. If a pint of milk is made up from milk powder, it must be stored in a refrigerator as soon as the water is added, to prevent any bacteria present from multiplying.

Foods containing salt and sugar absorb water, making it unavailable for bacterial growth.

Time

If bacteria are provided with food, water and a temperature near 37°C, they will divide into two approximately every 20 minutes. A few food-poisoning bacteria cannot cause illness but if food contaminated with bacteria is kept for a sufficiently long time in the right conditions the number of bacteria will increase, making the food poisonous. If food is eaten shortly after it is cooked or prepared, the risk of food poisoning is considerably reduced.

Summary

- ❏ The four requirements for bacterial growth are warmth, food, moisture and time.
- ❏ The bacteria which cause food poisoning grow best at 37°C.
- ❏ The temperature and humidity of the kitchen provide excellent conditions for the growth and multiplication of bacteria.
- ❏ Bacteria are not killed by the cold but most of those which cause food poisoning stop multiplying in a refrigerator.
- ❏ Bacteria grow best in foods which are high in moisture and are not too acid, not too sugary and not too salty.
- ❏ Bacteria cannot grow and multiply without moisture but they can remain dormant in dried foods.

4 FOOD CONTAMINATION

Food contamination can be biological (caused by bacteria, yeasts or moulds) or physical (caused by the presence of foreign bodies).

Bacterial contamination

Bacteria are present on and in raw meat, food handlers, animals, insects, soil, dust and refuse and any of these sources may be responsible for contaminating previously uncontaminated food.

Raw meat

Animals and poultry frequently carry pathogenic bacteria in their intestines. When the animals are slaughtered and dressed, these bacteria may spread over the surface of the meat where they will grow and multiply rapidly unless the meat is refrigerated immediately and kept under refrigeration during transport and storage in the butcher's shop. If these storage rules are observed the bacteria on contaminated meat will remain dormant but they will be able to grow and multiply again as soon as the meat is removed from refrigerated storage into normal room temperatures. However reputable the supplier, raw meat almost always carries pathogenic bacteria. These will normally be killed in the cooking process but care must be taken by the food handler not to let them have a chance to multiply and not to let them spread to foods which have already been cooked.

Food handlers

Pathogenic bacteria from food handlers can be spread into food, usually via the hands, during preparation and service. Everybody carries bacteria in their mouth, nose, intestines and on their skin and some of these bacteria will inevitably be transferred to food.

Carriers

A small percentage of the population are carriers of pathogenic bacteria and although they do not always have the symptoms of food poisoning, pathogenic bacteria are present in the intestinal tract and are therefore passed in their faeces. There are two types of carrier.

A *convalescent carrier* is someone who has recently recovered from food poisoning but is still harbouring pathogenic bacteria in the intestinal tract. A *healthy carrier* is someone who has not suffered from food poisoning but is nevertheless carrying pathogenic bacteria in the intestinal tract.

Convalescent and healthy carriers who fail to wash their hands after going to the toilet will contaminate the food they are preparing (*faecal–oral transmission*).

Animals and insects

Flies, rats, mice, birds, other insects and animals including pets frequently carry pathogenic bacteria in their intestines and on their feet and fur and must therefore not be allowed to come into contact with food or equipment which will be used for food preparation.

Soil, dust and refuse

Soil contains spores of some of the pathogenic bacteria. Raw vegetables must therefore always be cleaned thoroughly in a section of the kitchen used only for this purpose and then transferred to another section for further preparation.

Refuse and waste food should be placed in a bin immediately. Bins in food rooms should be emptied regularly.

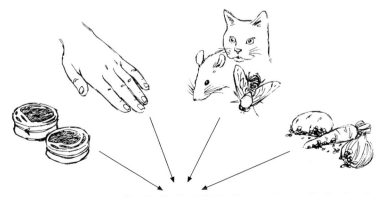

All these carry food-poisoning bacteria

Transfer of bacteria

Cross-contamination is the transfer of bacteria from a contaminated source to an uncontaminated food (usually freshly cooked food). Bacteria are not able to move from one food to another by themselves. They can be transferred directly or indirectly. Indirect contamination relies on other things to transfer bacteria from food to food (*vehicles of contamination*).

Examples of indirect contamination

1　Using a chopping board, a working surface or other kitchen equipment for the preparation of raw and cooked foods without washing it thoroughly between each use.

2　Using a knife or other utensil without washing it thoroughly between each use.

3　The hands of a food handler which are not washed in between preparing different types of food, e.g. raw and cooked meat, or after touching any source of bacteria, e.g. the nose, mouth, hair, pets.

Examples of direct contamination

1　Sneezing or coughing over food.

2　Incorrect positioning of foods in a refrigerator. For example, raw meat must always be placed below cooked food so that blood (which often contains pathogenic bacteria) cannot drip on to the cooked food.

Examples of cross-contamination

1　*A mincer which has been used for raw meat and then for cooked corned beef.* A chef working in a busy kitchen is making liver pâté. He minces the raw liver and decides to leave cleaning the mincer until he has got the pâté into the oven.

　　Before the first chef has finished the preparation of the pâté, a second chef uses the mincer for some cooked beef which is to be used for a rissole. In this way, some bacteria from the liver are transferred to the cooked beef.

　　The rissoles are left in the kitchen for several hours before they are cooked. During this time the bacteria increase to a sufficient number to cause food poisoning. As all the ingredients in the rissoles have already been cooked, they are only lightly browned before serving and the temperature reached in the centre of the rissoles during cooking is not sufficiently high to kill all the bacteria.

　　Vehicle of contamination: the mincer.

　　How food poisoning could have been prevented: by thoroughly washing the mincer immediately after use.

2 *A knife which has been used for cutting raw meat and not washed thoroughly before it is used for slicing cooked meat.* A chef is preparing sandwiches for a children's picnic. He has just finished cutting up raw meat for a casserole and as he is in a hurry he gives his knife a quick wipe on his overall and continues to use it to slice some ham.

A smear of blood from the raw meat is left on the knife and when the cooked ham is sliced with the same knife a few pathogenic bacteria are transferred to it. The ham is then used to make sandwiches.

It is a warm day and before the sandwiches are eaten the bacteria increase to sufficient numbers to cause food poisoning.

Vehicle of contamination: the knife.

How food poisoning could have been prevented: by using a different knife to cut the ham or by thoroughly washing the knife after using it for the raw meat and before using it for the cooked meat.

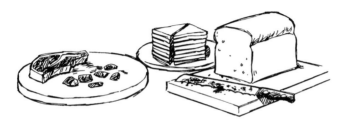

3 *A chef develops a heavy cold but does not report it to his employer and continues to work as usual on the preparation of desserts.* While piping cream on to a trifle the chef sneezes. He naturally turns away from the food and sneezes into his handkerchief but he does not wash his hands before continuing with his work. A few bacteria from the handkerchief are transferred to his hands and from there to the cream on the trifle. The trifle is put on the sweet trolley and most of it is eaten fairly quickly but two portions remain for several hours in the warm dining room. Those who ate the trifle at the beginning of the evening did not develop food poisoning but by the time the final two portions were eaten the bacteria had increased to a sufficient number to cause illness.

Vehicle of contamination: the hands.

How food poisoning could have been prevented: by washing his hands after touching the handkerchief. It is preferable to use disposable paper handkerchiefs which are destroyed after one use.

4 *Uncooked steak is placed on the top shelf of the refrigerator and uncovered roast chicken on the bottom shelf.* A drop of blood from the uncooked steak drips on to the uncovered roast chicken stored below it. A few pathogenic bacteria in the drop of blood are transferred to the chicken. They do not multiply in the refrigerator but remain dormant.

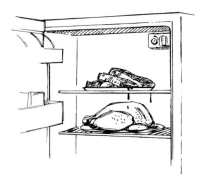

The chicken is served at a buffet on a warm afternoon. It is on display for three hours before it is eaten and during this time the bacteria increase to sufficient numbers to cause food poisoning.

Vehicle of contamination: the blood.

How food poisoning could have been prevented: by using different refrigerators for storing raw and cooked meat or by placing the uncooked steak at the bottom of the refrigerator and the cooked chicken at the top.

Colour coding of equipment

In order to avoid cross-contamination, equipment such as chopping boards and knives should be used for the preparation of only one type of food. A colour coding system (in which a small coloured tag is fixed to the equipment) is a way of identifying which equipment should be used for which type of food. Chopping boards in different colours are available.

Colour code	Equipment to be used only for:
Red	Raw meat and poultry
Green	Fruits and vegetables
Blue	Raw fish
Brown	Cooked meats
White	Dairy products

Physical contamination

Foreign bodies

Food can also be harmful due to the presence of foreign bodies. It is an offence under the Food Safety Act 1990 to sell a product contaminated with a foreign body.

The following list gives examples of items which have been found in food and the precautions necessary to minimise the risk of such contamination.

Foreign body	Prevention
Bolts, nuts, wire, oil and grease, flaking paint, cleaning chemicals 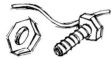	Maintain a high standard of cleanliness and decoration. Take care not to lose nuts, bolts, etc. from equipment during cleaning and maintenance work. Use food-grade lubricants
Cardboard, string, staples, paper, polythene, wood splinters 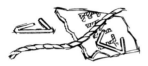	Do not unpack goods near open food. Ask suppliers to use adhesive tape rather than staples to fasten boxes
Earrings, false fingernails, buttons, pentops, hairs 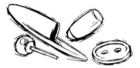	Wear suitable protective clothing when preparing food and do not carry pens, combs, etc. in the pockets. Do not wear jewellery except plain wedding rings
Sweet-papers, cigarette ends and matches 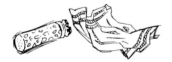	Do not smoke or eat when preparing food. Ensure self-service food is adequately protected from customers
Glass and china 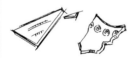	Do not use glass in a food preparation area unless it is unavoidable. Discard any food from a broken or chipped container
Cat, dog and animal hairs and feathers, rodent droppings, pest and insect bodies 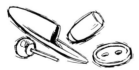	Do not allow animals in an industrial kitchen. Ensure it is kept free of pests by employing a reputable pest control contractor. Do not position electronic fly killers above open food
Bones from meat and fish, vegetable stalks and vegetables with imperfections due to poor trimming 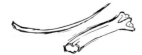	Prepare a written specification for permissible levels of contamination and agree this with supplier

Many systems are available for foreign body detection and removal such as sieves, X-ray and optical systems and metal detectors instead of or as well as human spotters. It is very important to ensure that any suppliers have installed suitable systems in their factories.

Any customer complaints concerning foreign bodies in food should be taken seriously and every effort made to identify the source of the contaminant. If necessary, the method of food preparation should be altered to prevent similar occurrences. Written evidence of the steps taken to minimise the risk of foreign body contamination would provide a due diligence defence in the event of a prosecution.

Summary

❑ The main sources of pathogenic bacteria in the kitchen are raw meat, food handlers, animals, insects, soil, dust and refuse.
❑ Cross-contamination is the transfer of bacteria from a contaminated source to uncontaminated food.
❑ Colour coding of equipment helps to prevent cross-contamination.
❑ Foreign bodies in food are a health hazard and may cause choking, cut mouths or food poisoning.

5 BACTERIAL FOOD POISONING AND FOOD-BORNE DISEASE

Bacterial food poisoning

The following bacteria frequently cause food poisoning:

❑ Salmonella (see p. 29)

❑ *Staphylococcus aureus* (see p. 35)

❑ *Clostridium perfringens* (see p. 40)

❑ *Bacillus cereus* (see p. 46).

The following bacteria cause food poisoning less frequently:

❑ *Clostridium botulinum* (see p. 57)

❑ Some strains of *Escherichia coli* (see p. 153).

All bacteria have two names. The *generic name* is written first and with a capital letter, e.g. *Clostridium*, *Bacillus*. The *specific name* is written with a small letter after the generic name, e.g. *perfringens*, *cereus*. Bacteria with the same generic name have similar characteristics, e.g. shape, oxygen requirements, enterotoxin production and spore formation.

There are approximately 2000 species of the Salmonella genus *(e.g. Salmonella typhimurium, Salmonella enteritidis, Salmonella hadar, Salmonella newport)* but since most of them cause food poisoning it is usual to talk about Salmonella food poisoning without distinguishing which species is actually the cause. Salmonella, *Staphylococcus aureus, Clostridium perfringens* and *Bacillus cereus* are all common causes of food poisoning in the UK and many other countries.

How many bacteria must be present to cause food poisoning?

Quite frequently we eat food which contains a few food-poisoning bacteria but small numbers of them do not cause illness. One million or more food-poisoning bacteria must be present before a healthy adult will feel any harmful effects. A child under one year, an old person or a sick person would be affected by the presence of far fewer bacteria. Special care must therefore be taken when preparing food for people in these categories.

Food poisoning is occasionally fatal. The deaths caused by food poisoning are usually in very young babies or in old or severely ill people.

Incubation period

This is the time that passes between the entry of the poisonous food into the body and the occurrence of the first symptoms. The length of the incubation period helps to decide which type of bacteria has caused the food poisoning. Some types of bacteria cause food poisoning with a relatively long incubation period (up to two days) and other types of bacteria cause food poisoning with a relatively short incubation period (two hours). The length of the incubation period also depends on the number of bacteria present as well as the type of bacteria causing the food poisoning. If the food is very heavily contaminated with a certain type of bacteria, the incubation period will be shorter than if the food is contaminated with only half the number of the same type of bacteria.

Duration

The duration of the illness is the time between the appearance of the first symptoms of food poisoning and the clearing up of the last ones. This is rarely longer than three days and may be as short as a few hours. When all the symptoms of food poisoning have gone, it does not necessarily mean that there are no harmful bacteria in the intestinal tract (see Convalescent carriers, p. 19).

Food-borne disease

The following bacteria cause food-borne diseases:

❏   Campylobacter (see p. 51)

❏   *E. coli* 0157 (see p. 54)

❏   *Salmonella typhi* (see p. 153)

❏   *Salmonella paratyphi* (see p. 154)

❏   Shigella (see p. 58)

❏   *Listeria monocytogenes* (see p. 58).

Bacterial food-borne diseases can be caused by the ingestion of small numbers of particularly harmful bacteria. Any type of food or water can transmit the pathogenic bacteria to the sufferer. Multiplication need not take place. The symptoms of food-borne disease vary widely and may or may not include vomiting and diarrhoea. In some cases rashes, septicaemia and kidney failure are the main symptoms.

Food-borne diseases are frequently transmitted by:

❏   contaminated drinking water and ice

❏   food such as salads and fruits which has been washed in contaminated water

❏   shellfish or watercress gathered from contaminated water

❏   dehydrated food which has been rehydrated with contaminated water

❏   food handlers with poor standards of personal hygiene (faecal–oral transmission).

After a natural disaster such as an earthquake or flooding, the drinking water sometimes becomes contaminated with sewage, causing large outbreaks of these diseases.

How many bacteria must be present to cause illness?

Very small numbers of bacteria compared with the large numbers needed to cause food poisoning. As few as 100 bacterial cells may be sufficient to cause a food-borne disease.

Incubation period

The incubation period is very variable and may be anything from one to 21 days.

Duration

The duration of food-borne diseases is very variable and may be anything from one day to several months. Sometimes the patient may suffer permanent damage; for example, *E. coli* 0157 can cause kidney failure.

DIFFERENCES BETWEEN BACTERIAL FOOD POISONING AND FOOD-BORNE DISEASES	
Bacterial food poisoning	**Bacterial food-borne diseases**
Large numbers of the bacteria or the toxin produced by them are ingested	Relatively small numbers of the bacteria cause illness
Bacterial multiplication in food is an essential feature of food poisoning	Bacterial multiplication does not necessarily take place
Caused only by food	May be caused by food or water or spread by other means such as person to person
The incubation period is relatively short: 2–36 hours	The incubation period is relatively long: 1–21 days
Symptoms: vomiting and/or diarrhoea	Symptoms: a wide variety, not necessarily vomiting and diarrhoea

6 SALMONELLA

Salmonella is a short, rod-shaped bacterium.

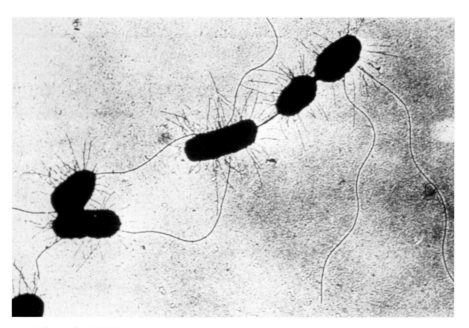

Salmonella × 5000 approx.

People can be severely ill with Salmonella food poisoning and it is occasionally fatal, in elderly, very young or sick people.

Type of food poisoning

Salmonella causes infective food poisoning.

Large numbers of living bacteria must be present in the food when it is eaten. Some of them will be destroyed by the acid in the stomach but some will be protected by food and pass through to the small intestine where the near-neutral conditions allow them to multiply. As they increase in numbers, some of the cells die and release a poisonous substance which causes fever, diarrhoea and vomiting. Since it takes some time for the bacteria to increase in numbers to a level which causes symptoms, the incubation period is relatively long.

Incubation period	12–72 hours
Duration of illness	1–8 days
Symptoms	Fever, headache, abdominal pains, diarrhoea and vomiting

Natural origin of Salmonella

1   Salmonella is found in the intestines of many farm animals, particularly poultry, It is therefore present on raw meat.

2   Mice, rats, domestic pets, flies and birds also often carry Salmonella in their intestines and on their fur and feet.

Means of access to food

1   Brought into the kitchen on or in foods of animal origin, e.g. poultry, meat, unpasteurised milk, dried egg powder.

Salmonella is normally present only on the surface of raw meat but is often present in the central cavity of poultry or in the centre of minced meat products such as sausages and hamburgers. These foods may cause poisoning if they are inadequately cooked or they may contaminate other goods which have already been cooked.

Unpasteurised milk is sometimes contaminated with Salmonella. Pasteurisation destroys Salmonella.

Duck eggs frequently harbour Salmonella and some hen eggs do but it is thought to be only a small proportion. The shell of both types may be contaminated with Salmonella.

2   Insects, birds, vermin and domestic pets can spread Salmonella into food if they are allowed to be present in the kitchen.

3   People working in the kitchen are sometimes, unknown to them, carrying Salmonella in their intestines and may contaminate food if they don't wash their hands after a visit to the toilet.

Destruction

Salmonella is readily killed by heat. It does not form a spore.

Foods usually involved

Foods causing this type of food poisoning have either been cooked inadequately or have been contaminated after cooking, e.g. poultry which has not been properly defrosted, cold meats which have been contaminated from raw meat.

Preventive measures

1   Thaw frozen food completely before cooking. Allow 24 hours to thaw a 3 lb (1.5 kg) chicken in the refrigerator. A large turkey would take too long to thaw in a refrigerator and should be thawed in a chiller or a cool area of the kitchen.

2   Cook food thoroughly, making sure the temperature at the centre of the food is high enough to kill bacteria. Where possible, stir to avoid cool spots, especially when cooking by microwave.

3   Use different surfaces and equipment, e.g. chopping boards, knives, etc., for preparing raw food and cooked food.

4   Clean and disinfect all equipment thoroughly after each use.

5   Store raw and cooked foods (particularly meat) separately.

6   Wash hands after handling raw meat, poultry and eggs.

7   Wash hands after using the toilet.

8   Keep food as cold as possible to prevent multiplication of Salmonella.

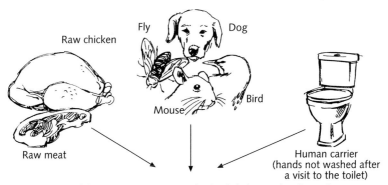

Raw chicken   Fly   Dog

Mouse   Bird

Raw meat   Human carrier
(hands not washed after
a visit to the toilet)

Any of these may contaminate the foods below with Salmonella

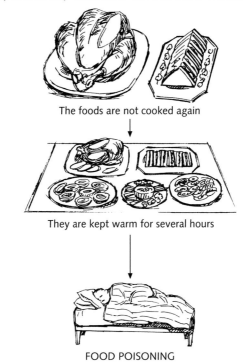

The foods are not cooked again

They are kept warm for several hours

FOOD POISONING

A typical chain of events leading to food poisoning by Salmonella

Roast chicken was a favourite on the menu at a restaurant where many people had their midday meal. Normally the chickens were taken from the freezer the previous evening and left to defrost in the refrigerator overnight.

One evening the chef forgot to remove the chickens from the deep freeze so he arrived at work early the next morning and put them in a sink of hot water for two hours. He than ran some hot water inside the chicken carcasses and managed to melt some of the ice. He hastily stuffed the chickens and put them into the oven to cook for lunchtime, thinking that the rest of the ice would melt in the heat of the oven.

After the normal cooking time he was relieved to find that the flesh appeared to be perfectly cooked and so he served it at lunchtime as usual with a portion of stuffing.

The following day several people in the area had to go to their doctors with severe headaches, abdominal pains, diarrhoea and vomiting. They were questioned about where they had eaten their meals during the last 36 hours and an outbreak of Salmonella food poisoning was traced to the restaurant where the chickens were served.

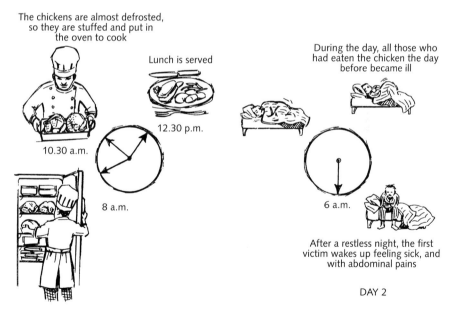

The chickens are almost defrosted, so they are stuffed and put in the oven to cook

Lunch is served

During the day, all those who had eaten the chicken the day before became ill

12.30 p.m.

10.30 a.m.

8 a.m.

6 a.m.

After a restless night, the first victim wakes up feeling sick, and with abdominal pains

DAY 2

Chef arrives early to remove the chickens from the freezer

DAY 1

Fault

Frozen meat, particularly poultry, must be thawed completely before commencing cooking. If ice is present in the centre of the chicken, a great deal of heat is used to melt it. It will take far longer for the internal temperature to equal the external temperature than it would if the chicken were completely defrosted. Even if the chicken is cooked for the recommended time, the temperature in the centre of the bird at the end of the cooking time is not sufficiently high to kill Salmonella but is probably an optimum temperature for its multiplication. It is advisable to cook stuffing separately and not in the bird, where it will slow down heat penetration.

7 STAPHYLOCOCCUS AUREUS

Staphylococcus aureus is a round bacterium.

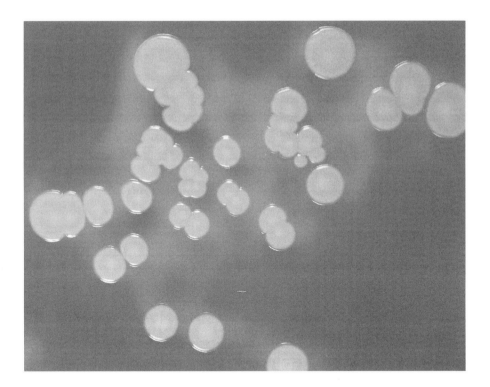

Staphylococcus aureus × 6400 approx.

The symptoms of food poisoning caused by *Staphylococcus aureus* are severe for a short period of time but the illness is rarely fatal.

Type of food poisoning

Staphylococcus aureus causes toxic food poisoning. Whilst growing and multiplying in food stored at a warm temperature, it produces a toxin (a poisonous substance). When the food is swallowed the toxin irritates the stomach lining, causing vomiting. The incubation period is therefore relatively short and the main symptom is vomiting.

Incubation period	1–7 hours (usually 2–4 hours)
Duration of illness	6–24 hours
Symptoms	Vomiting, sometimes abdominal pains and diarrhoea

Natural origin of *Staphylococcus aureus*

Staphylococcus aureus is frequently present in the human nose and throat and on the skin of healthy people. It is known as a *commensal* because it is completely harmless when present in these areas. It is found also in large numbers in boils, styes and septic cuts.

　　Staphylococcus aureus is sometimes present in unpasteurised milk.

Means of access to food

1　People working in the kitchen who sneeze or cough over food or who have septic cuts, boils, styes, etc. and do not cover them with an adequate waterproof dressing.

2　Unpasteurised milk and products made from unpasteurised milk which are not cooked or only lightly cooked.

Destruction

Staphylococcus aureus does not form a spore and is therefore readily killed by heat (1–2 minutes in boiling water) BUT the toxin which it produces in food is more resistant to heat than the bacterial cell and can withstand up to 30 minutes in boiling water. It is therefore possible for lightly cooked food to contain active toxin but no live bacteria. This food will still cause food poisoning.

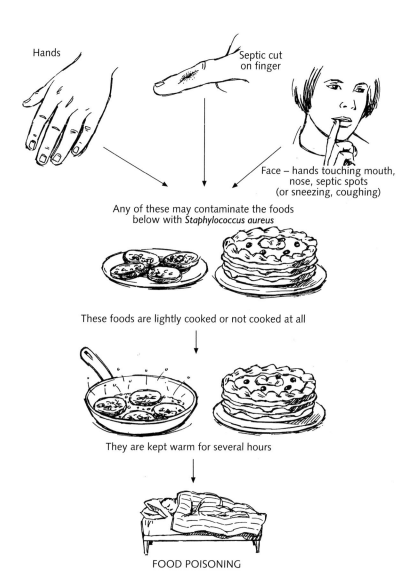

Hands

Septic cut on finger

Face – hands touching mouth, nose, septic spots (or sneezing, coughing)

Any of these may contaminate the foods below with *Staphylococcus aureus*

These foods are lightly cooked or not cooked at all

They are kept warm for several hours

FOOD POISONING

Foods usually involved

Foods causing *Staphylococcus aureus* food poisoning are usually those which have been contaminated by the food handler after they have been cooked and are then eaten cold or after an inadequate reheating process, e.g. sliced cold meats, cream dishes, custards and other milk products and stuffed rolled joints which have not been cooked through to the centre. Staphylococcus is able to grow in higher concentrations of salt than the other food-poisoning bacteria and therefore outbreaks involving salty foods, e.g. ham, are often traced to Staphylococcus.

Preventive measures

1   Maintain a high standard of personal hygiene.
2   Handle food as little as possible. Always use serving tongs for food which will not be heated again.
3   Keep food covered.
4   Keep food as cold as possible to prevent the multiplication of *Staphylococcus aureus*.

A typical chain of events leading to food poisoning by *Staphylococcus aureus*

At a school canteen, custard is served most days with the pudding. As it is fairly easy to prepare, a new member of staff was allocated this task. He starts work at 8.00 am and on one particular morning as there is no other urgent work, he starts by preparing the custard. At 8.30 am he moves on to another task and leaves the custard to cool but suddenly wonders if he remembered to add the sugar. He tastes it with a spoon and thinks it seems sweet enough but just checks it again using the same spoon without washing it. He is then quite satisfied that the sugar has been added. The custard is left in the kitchen for the rest of the morning and at 12.15 pm it is warmed up and served for lunch at 12.30 pm.

That afternoon several children start to feel sick and have acute stomach pains. By 5.30 p.m. that evening many of the children who had eaten the custard are ill and an outbreak of food poisoning caused by *Staphylococcus aureus* is confirmed.

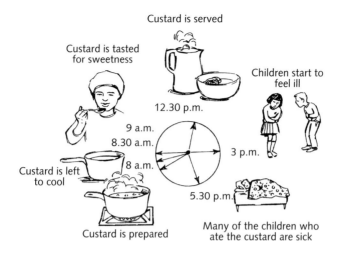

Custard is served

Custard is tasted for sweetness

Children start to feel ill

12.30 p.m.

9 a.m.

8.30 a.m.

3 p.m.

Custard is left to cool

8 a.m.

5.30 p.m.

Custard is prepared

Many of the children who ate the custard are sick

Fault

A spoon which has been put into the mouth must never be returned to food without first washing it. *Staphylococcus aureus* can be transferred from the mouth to food via the spoon. If the food is left for some time at a warm temperature the bacteria will grow, multiply and produce toxins. If the food is reheated inadequately the exotoxin will not be destroyed.

8 *CLOSTRIDIUM PERFRINGENS*

Clostridium perfringens is a rod-shaped bacterium. It can form a spore when conditions are unfavourable for growth and is also an anaerobe so grows in the absence of oxygen.

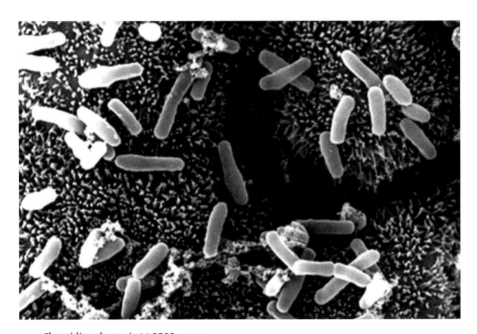

Clostridium bacteria × 3200 approx.

Clostridium perfringens food poisoning is rarely fatal.

Type of food poisoning

Clostridium perfringens does not produce toxin when it is multiplying in food stored at a warm temperature but when that food is eaten the bacteria form spores and at the same time an endotoxin, which irritates the intestinal wall, causing diarrhoea. This is not exactly the same as toxic food poisoning or infective food poisoning but has some characteristics of both. The incubation period is longer than with food poisoning where exotoxin has been produced, as caused by *Staphylococcus aureus*, and shorter than infective food poisoning, as caused by Salmonella.

Incubation period	8–22 hours (usually 12–18 hours)
Duration of illness	12–24 hours
Symptoms	Abdominal pains and diarrhoea. The patient rarely vomits

Natural origin of *Clostridium perfringens*

1   *C. perfringens* is frequently present in human and animal intestines.

2   Flies and bluebottles are usually heavily infected with *C. perfringens*.

3   Spores of *C. perfringens* are found in soil.

Means of access to food

1   Brought into the kitchen on raw meat. The meat itself may cause food poisoning since *C. perfringens* can survive cooking processes by forming a spore. Bacteria from the raw meat may also be transferred to cooked foods in careless preparation.

2   Vegetables coated with soil or dust from sacks or packing cases may contaminate foods with *C. perfringens* if the soil or dust settles on food.

3   People working in the kitchen may be carrying *C. perfringens* in their intestines and may spread the bacteria into food if their hands are not washed after a visit to the toilet.

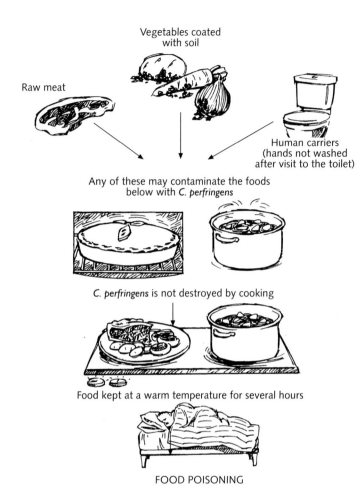

Vegetables coated with soil

Raw meat

Human carriers (hands not washed after visit to the toilet)

Any of these may contaminate the foods below with *C. perfringens*

C. perfringens is not destroyed by cooking

Food kept at a warm temperature for several hours

FOOD POISONING

Destruction

The spores of *C. perfringens* are not destroyed by normal cooking methods. They can withstand boiling, steaming, stewing or braising for up to four hours. The spores do not multiply but if the food is cooled slowly and kept warm for some time before serving, the spores germinate, producing vegetative bacteria which multiply rapidly.

Foods usually involved

C. perfringens does not grow readily in the presence of oxygen. It is most frequently found reproducing rapidly at the bottom of a lukewarm meat casserole or stock pot or at the centre of large food masses where there is little air (oxygen), e.g. meat pies, minced meat dishes. Reheated meat dishes are also frequently a cause of *C. perfringens* food poisoning since the spore it forms will survive each reheating process.

Most outbreaks involve a large number of people because *C. perfringens* is more commonly found in foods that have been prepared in bulk.

Preventive measures

1   Use separate preparation areas for raw food (especially meat and vegetables) and cooked food and remove dirt and waste regularly from them.

2   Cool cooked foods rapidly and refrigerate promptly. To do this it may be necessary to break up large volumes of meat and cool and store it in separate smaller containers. Large joints of meat should be removed from the cooking liquor immediately after cooking to speed up cooling.

3   Use different surfaces and equipment, e.g. chopping boards, knives, etc., for preparing raw and cooked food.

4   Clean all equipment thoroughly after each use.

5   Store raw foods (particularly meat and unwashed vegetables) away from cooked food.

6   Wash hands after handling raw meat and unwashed vegetables.

7   If reheating of food is necessary, it must be reheated rapidly and thoroughly and then served quickly. Meat products should not be reheated more than once.

A typical chain of events leading to food poisoning by *Clostridium perfringens*

The staff in a works canteen are responsible for preparing a main meal for all the people at the factory. There are two shifts. The early shift eats lunch at 11.00 am. The late shift eats at 2.00 pm.

One day, one of the dishes on the menu is beef casserole. The chef preparing the casserole gathers together the ingredients (beef, onions, carrots and swedes) and takes them to the working surface where he usually does his preparation. He cuts the beef and puts it on one side and then scrapes the vegetables, chops them and puts everything together in the casserole which is then cooked in time for the first shift. It is taken from the oven a few minutes before 11.00 am and served piping hot to the people on the first shift. However, not all of it is used so rather than see it wasted, the chef decides to leave it in the warming cabinet to keep it warm for the second shift. The temperature in the warming cabinet is 45°C.

That night some of the people from the factory start to feel ill with severe abdominal pains and diarrhoea. An outbreak of food poisoning caused by *C. perfringens* is confirmed and traced to the beef casserole although it is only the people on the second shift who are ill and none of those from the first shift are affected.

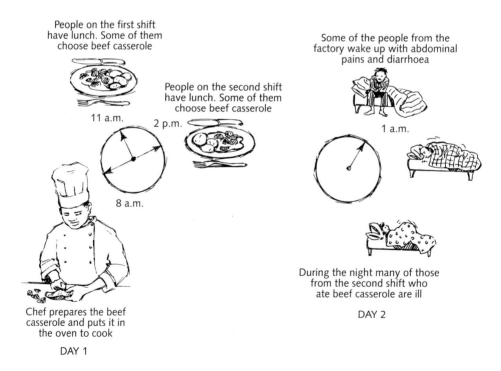

People on the first shift have lunch. Some of them choose beef casserole

11 a.m.

2 p.m.

People on the second shift have lunch. Some of them choose beef casserole

8 a.m.

Chef prepares the beef casserole and puts it in the oven to cook

DAY 1

Some of the people from the factory wake up with abdominal pains and diarrhoea

1 a.m.

During the night many of those from the second shift who ate beef casserole are ill

DAY 2

Faults

1   Separate working areas, equipment and utensils should be used for preparing raw meat and vegetables.

2   Foods which are suitable for bacterial growth should never be kept warm. If they are not served immediately they must be kept hot, at a temperature above 63°C, or cold, at a temperature below 5°C. In this case the casserole was kept warm for three hours in between servings. *C. perfringens* from either the raw meat or from soil on the vegetables had survived the cooking process by forming spores which were able to germinate, grow and multiply rapidly when the casserole was kept at a temperature of 45°C.

9 *BACILLUS CEREUS*

Bacillus cereus is a rod-shaped bacterium. It can form a spore when conditions are unfavourable for growth. It is an aerobe and therefore requires oxygen for growth.

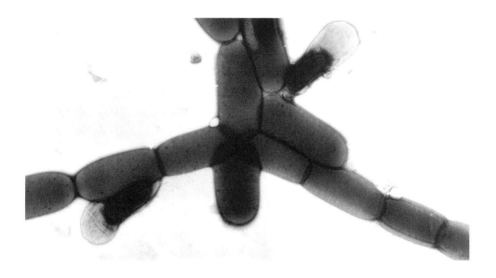

Bacillus cereus × 5000

The onset of symptoms of *Bacillus cereus* food poisoning can be very sudden but it is usually over fairly quickly. It is most unlikely to be fatal.

Type of food poisoning

Bacillus cereus usually causes toxic food poisoning. Whilst *B. cereus* is growing and multiplying in food stored at a warm temperature, it produces an exotoxin. When the food is swallowed the exotoxin irritates the stomach lining, causing vomiting.

Incubation period	1–5 hours
Duration	6–24 hours
Symptoms	Vomiting, abdominal pains, occasionally diarrhoea

There is a second type of *B. cereus* food poisoning which is rare in the United Kingdom. Toxins are produced in the intestine but not in the food before it is eaten. The incubation period is longer and the main symptom is diarrhoea.

Natural origin of *Bacillus cereus*

Bacillus cereus is found in the soil and in dust.

Means of access to food

The spores of *B. cereus* are brought into the kitchen on cereals, particularly rice. Cornflour and spices are also often contaminated.

Destruction

The spores of *B. cereus* are not easily destroyed by heat and will survive most cooking processes. They do not multiply but if the food is cooled slowly or kept warm for some time before serving, they will germinate, producing vegetative bacteria which multiply rapidly at these temperatures and produce a very heat-resistant toxin. Subsequent reheating is unlikely to destroy the exotoxin.

Foods usually involved

Reheated rice is almost always the cause of *B. cereus* food poisoning.

Preventive measures

1   Cool cooked food rapidly and refrigerate promptly.

2   If reheating of the food is necessary, it must be reheated rapidly and thoroughly and then served quickly. Never reheat rice more than once.

A typical chain of events leading to food poisoning by *Bacillus cereus*

A student has invited 12 friends to come for a curry after a football match. He has planned to cook a curry and serve it with plain boiled rice. He knows he will not have time to prepare the curry on the evening of the party so he prepares it on the previous evening and after cooking it he cools it quickly and puts it in the refrigerator to store overnight. He also cooks the rice the night before but as there is no room in the refrigerator he covers it and leaves it on the working surface in the kitchen thinking that rice is a 'safe' food anyway.

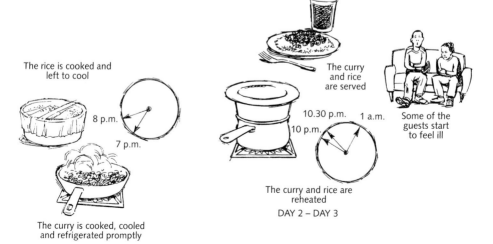

The rice is cooked and left to cool

8 p.m.

7 p.m.

The curry is cooked, cooled and refrigerated promptly

DAY 1

The curry and rice are served

10.30 p.m.   1 a.m.

10 p.m.

Some of the guests start to feel ill

The curry and rice are reheated

DAY 2 – DAY 3

The next evening, when they return from the football, he reheats the curry thoroughly and then warms the rice over a pan of boiling water and serves both to his friends.

Even before the evening is over, several of the friends suddenly start to feel very sick and some of the others are ill during the night. An outbreak of food poisoning due to *B. cereus* is traced to the rice.

Fault

Bacteria which had survived the first cooking of the rice by forming spores had germinated into vegetative bacteria, multiplied and produced toxin during long slow cooling overnight. The rice was not reheated sufficiently to destroy the toxin in it.

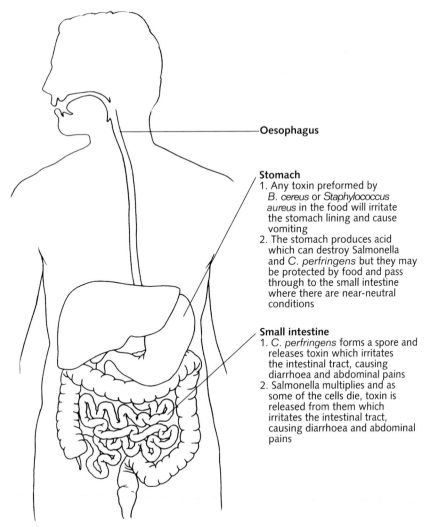

Oesophagus

Stomach
1. Any toxin preformed by *B. cereus* or *Staphylococcus aureus* in the food will irritate the stomach lining and cause vomiting
2. The stomach produces acid which can destroy Salmonella and *C. perfringens* but they may be protected by food and pass through to the small intestine where there are near-neutral conditions

Small intestine
1. *C. perfringens* forms a spore and releases toxin which irritates the intestinal tract, causing diarrhoea and abdominal pains
2. Salmonella multiplies and as some of the cells die, toxin is released from them which irritates the intestinal tract, causing diarrhoea and abdominal pains

The human digestive system

THE BACTERIA WHICH COMMONLY CAUSE FOOD POISONING

	Salmonella	Staphylococcus	C. perfringens	B. cereus
Incubation period	12–72 hours	1–7 hours	8–22 hours	1-5 hours
Duration of illness	1–8 days	6–24 hours	12–24 hours	6–24 hours
Means of access to the kitchen	Poultry and other raw meat. Animals. Human carriers	Mainly through humans, from the nose, mouth, infected wounds and sores	Raw meat. Dust, soil, flies. Human carriers	Cereals, especially rice
Foods usually involved	Meat and meat products	Almost any food which has been handled and not cooked or only lightly cooked afterwards, e.g. sliced cold meats, cream and milk products	Meat dishes, e.g. stews, pies, gravy, meat stock	Rice
Destruction	Vegetative bacteria readily destroyed by heat. Does not form spores. Does not produce a toxin	Vegetative bacteria readily destroyed by heat. Does not form spores. Exotoxin destroyed by boiling for 30 mins	Forms spores which can survive several hours in boiling water. Therefore not normally destroyed in cooking processes	Forms spores which can survive several hours in boiling water. Therefore not normally destroyed in cooking processes

10 CAMPYLO-BACTER

Campylobacter jejuni and *Campylobacter coli* are the most common causes of diarrhoea in the UK.

CAMPYLOBACTER SPECIES: LABORATORY REPORTS 1991–99								
Year	1991	1992	1993	1994	1995	1996	1997	1998	1999
No. of cases	32 636	38 552	39 422	44 414	43 876	43 337	50 177	58 059	54 994

Source: PHLS

The presence of 500 bacterial cells or less is sufficient to cause this disease.

Incubation period	1–11 days (usually 2–5)
Duration	2–5 days
Symptoms	Abdominal pain and profuse diarrhoea (usually bloodstained). Vomiting is rare

Natural origin of Campylobacter

Campylobacter naturally occur in the gastrointestinal tract of birds, cattle and domestic pets.

Means of access to food

1   Brought into the kitchen on poultry and raw meat which may contaminate cooked foods in careless preparation.

2   Unpasteurised milk and milk pecked by birds (usually magpies) on the doorstep.

3   Domestic pets in the kitchen can contaminate food and/or work surfaces.

4   Untreated water.

Destruction

Campylobacter does not form a spore and is destroyed by thorough cooking. It grows and multiplies most rapidly at warm temperatures (between 37°C and 43°C). It will not grow in food at normal room temperature and hence the food is used only as a means of transporting the bacteria into the body.

Foods usually involved

1   Raw and inadequately processed milk and 'pecked' milk.

2   Foods that have been cross-contaminated from raw meat and poultry.

Non-food causes of illness

Direct contact with infected pets and farm animals. The animals themselves are usually suffering from diarrhoea.

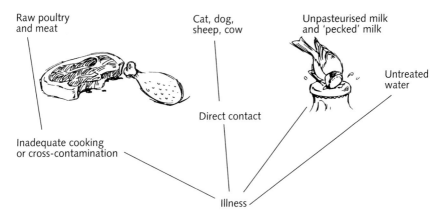

Causes of Campylobacter infection

Preventive measures

Because of the low infective dose, any breakdown in hygiene standards could potentially cause illness.

1   Use only sealed pasteurised milk and treated water in food preparation.

2   Keep pets out of food preparation areas.

3   Avoid cross-contamination from raw meat and poultry to cooked foods.

4   Thorough cooking.

11 *ESCHERICHIA COLI*

Escherichia coli (E. coli) are small rod-shaped bacteria.

Most types of *E. coli* bacteria are harmless and are sometimes present in large numbers in the human digestive tract. A few strains, not normally encountered in the UK, are responsible for the 'traveller's diarrhoea' which people sometimes suffer from when they first arrive in a foreign country.

One particular strain, known as *E. coli* 0157, produces a very harmful toxin and causes serious illness and even death, particularly in young children and the elderly.

The presence of 100 or less *E. coli* 0157 cells is sufficient to cause illness. In 1996 an outbreak in Scotland linked to a butcher's shop resulted in 500 cases, with 21 deaths.

E. COLI: LABORATORY REPORTS 1991–99								
Year	1992	1993	1994	1995	1996	1997	1998	1999
No. of cases	470	385	411	792	660	1087	890	1084

Source: PHLS

Incubation period	1–14 days (usually 3–4 days)
Duration	Two weeks or more. Some cases are fatal
Symptoms	Acute abdominal pain, bloody diarrhoea, kidney damage. *E. coli* 0157 is the main cause of kidney failure in children in the UK

Natural origin of *E. coli* 0157

The gastrointestinal tract of farm animals, especially cattle and possibly domestic pets.

Means of access to food

1   Brought into the kitchen on raw meat which may contaminate cooked foods in careless preparation.

2   Unpasteurised milk.

3   Untreated water.

Destruction

E. coli 0157 is not heat resistant and will be destroyed by normal cooking methods.

Foods usually involved

1   Inadequately cooked foods, particularly minced beef products. Undercooked beefburgers have often caused this illness. Great care must be taken when barbecuing beefburgers to ensure that the meat in the centre of the burger is thoroughly cooked. The juices should run clear and there should be no pink meat in the centre.

2   Any food which has been cross-contaminated from raw meat.

3   Unpasteurised milk and cheese made from it.

4   Unwashed raw vegetables.

Non-food causes of illness

1   Direct contact with animals, particularly cattle. There is a risk associated with visitors, especially children, to farm centres. The animals show no symptoms of illness.

2   Person-to-person spread (faecal–oral route), particularly in families, nurseries and infant schools.

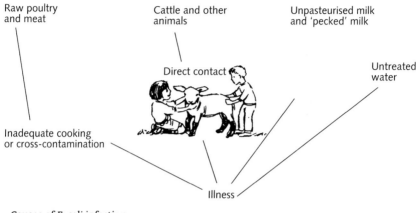

Causes of *E. coli* infection

Preventive measures

1   Avoid cross-contamination from raw meat to cooked foods. Use colour-coded chopping boards and knives. Clean and disinfect kitchen equipment after use.

2   Thorough cooking of food, particularly minced beef products.

3   Use only sealed pasteurised milk and treated water in food preparation.

4   Keep domestic pets out of food preparation areas.

12 FURTHER CAUSES OF FOOD POISONING AND FOOD-BORNE DISEASE

A few cases of food poisoning and food-borne disease are recorded each year that are attributed to causes other than those already described. They may be caused by different types of bacteria, viruses, chemicals or vegetable matter.

Bacteria

Clostridium botulinum

Clostridium botulinum food poisoning is very rare in the UK but because many of the cases that occur are fatal, great efforts are made to avoid causing this type of food poisoning.

Clostridium botulinum causes toxic food poisoning. The toxin is produced by the bacteria when they are growing in food under strictly anaerobic conditions (a complete absence of oxygen). These anaerobic conditions exist in canned food (see p. 128).

Botulinum toxin is a highly poisonous substance and people have died after eating only a mouthful of infected food. The symptoms are giddiness, double vision, headache, nausea and vomiting. The central nervous system is affected and paralysis of the respiratory tract is the usual cause of death.

Clostridium botulinum is found in soil and therefore on vegetables. It is also found in fish caught in some areas, notably the waters around Japan. It can produce a spore which will survive ordinary cooking methods but the toxin produced by it is not heat resistant and will usually be destroyed by boiling for a few minutes.

Most cases of botulism (food poisoning caused by *C. botulinum*) have occurred after eating understerilised canned food or food in faulty cans which has been contaminated after sterilisation. Food manufacturers take great care that all *C. botulinum* spores are destroyed in processing and only very rarely have commercially canned foods been the cause of this type of food poisoning. In the United States some people can their own vegetables and this has sometimes caused botulism. A Japanese delicacy, raw fermented fish, has also caused outbreaks of botulism.

Bacillary dysentery

Bacillary dysentery is a food-borne disease caused by a bacterium called Shigella. The incubation period is between one and seven days and the symptoms are severe diarrhoea, fever and sometimes vomiting.

Bacillary dysentery is spread by the faecal–oral route (transfer of bacteria from the faeces of infected people). Outbreaks in the UK sometimes occur in schools and nurseries as a result of contact with contaminated toilet seats and tap handles or lack of supervised hand washing. They may involve large numbers of children. It is a common illness in many countries, particularly those with poor sanitation. Dysentery can be controlled by strict attention to personal hygiene, taking great care to wash the hands after going to the toilet and before touching food.

Listeria monocytogenes

Cases of illness attributed to *Listeria monocytogenes* are relatively rare but these bacteria have attracted a lot of media attention, partly because the illness they cause can be serious or even fatal and partly because they are one of the few types of pathogenic bacteria that can grow at refrigeration temperatures.

Listeria monocytogenes is found widely distributed in the environment and is present in the intestines of many domestic and wild animals, including chickens, sheep and cattle. The bacteria can be passed into the milk of infected animals.

The vast majority of people who eat food contaminated with *Listeria monoocytogenes* will be unaffected or may at worst have a mild fever for a short time. However, two groups of people are particularly at risk of severe illness: pregnant women and sick people whose illness or treatment affects their immune system. Listeriosis in pregnant women can cause miscarriage or result in a stillbirth. In very young babies and in immunosuppressed patients, listeriosis can give rise to meningitis and septicaemia.

Foods that have frequently been found to contain Listeria and should therefore be avoided by vulnerable people include soft ripened cheese, for example Brie and Camembert, pâté, cook-chill meals (see p. 94), coleslaw and other prepacked salads in dressings, salami and continental sausages.

Viruses

Small round structured viruses (SRSVs) frequently cause diarrhoea and projectile vomiting. Viruses only multiply in living tissue and cannot multiply in food, which merely acts as a means of transport. Any type of food can therefore be involved.

The incubation period is usually 1–2 days and patients are infectious for a further two days after the symptoms have gone.

The infective dose is extremely low and person-to-person spread via the faecal–oral route is very common. The virus may also be airborne from infected vomit. Outbreaks of viral food poisoning often occur in schools and families because of the ease of transfer of the virus.

Viruses are destroyed by the temperatures reached in normal cooking methods and so viral food poisoning is usually transmitted by food which has not been cooked or has been handled after cooking by someone who is a carrier of the virus.

The polio virus can also be transmitted by food.

Chemical food poisoning

This type of food poisoning is relatively rare. It is caused as a result of contamination by chemicals during the growth, preparation, storage or cooking of the food. The symptoms are usually vomiting, diarrhoea and burning sensations within a hour (often a few minutes) of eating the food. In some instances chemicals build up in the body over a period of time, causing severe illness.

Most cases of chemical food poisoning are caused by carelessness in the home or an industrial establishment. Cleaning materials should be stored away from food and in such a way that they will not spill or leak from their containers. They must be clearly labelled and should never be decanted into food or drink containers.

There have been a few outbreaks of zinc poisoning due to the use of galvanised equipment with acid foods. Chipped enamel vessels can cause antimony poisoning, particularly if used with acid foods such as rhubarb, citrus fruits, apple and tomatoes.

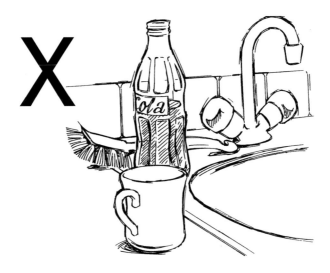

Insecticidal sprays, pesticides, food additives and packaging materials are all potential sources of chemical food poisoning but there are strict regulations for food producers and food manufacturers governing their use.

Poisonous plants and fungi

Certain plants naturally contain substances which are poisonous to human beings, for example toadstools, hemlock, deadly nightshade, rhubarb leaves. The most common cause of vegetable food poisoning is the toadstool which can easily be mistaken for a mushroom. The consumption of raw or undercooked red kidney beans causes severe vomiting. The naturally occurring poison present in raw red kidney beans can be destroyed by boiling them for 10 minutes. Canned red kidney beans are quite safe to eat without further cooking.

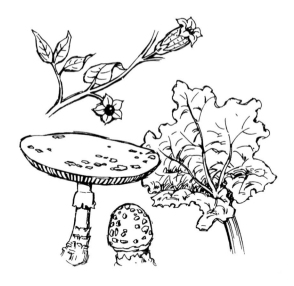

Summary

- ❏ Illness caused by *Clostridium botulinum*, Shigella or Listeria is relatively rare but the symptoms are severe and the illness may be fatal.
- ❏ Some viruses cause diarrhoea and vomiting.
- ❏ Certain chemicals, fungi and plants are known to cause food poisoning.

13 PERSONAL AND KITCHEN HYGIENE

Prevention of food poisoning

There are two aspects to the prevention of food poisoning.

1   A food handler must as far as possible prevent bacteria from entering food by maintaining a high standard of personal hygiene and by being aware of all possible sources of contamination in the kitchen.

2   A food handler must discourage the multiplication of any bacteria which may be present so that the numbers never become sufficiently large to cause an outbreak of food poisoning. This can be done by preparing, cooking and storing foods correctly (see Chapter 14).

Prevention of food-borne diseases

The multiplication of bacteria in food often does not occur in food-borne diseases. High standards of personal hygiene and care to avoid cross-contamination are therefore essential to prevent these diseases.

Hand washing

Pathogenic bacteria carried on the hands and transferred into food during its preparation are one of the most common causes of food contamination.

In all catering establishments, by law, there must be sufficient wash basins in places where the food handlers can reach them quickly and easily from where they are working. Wash basins and nail brushes must also be provided near the toilets. Wash hand-basins should not be used for food washing and hands should not be washed in sinks used for the preparation of food or for washing up.

Before commencing food preparation, hands and forearms should always be washed with hot water and soap and not just rinsed under the tap.

A liquid soap dispenser is more hygienic than a soap tablet which is used by everybody. Some soaps are called *bactericidal* soaps because they contain a disinfectant which helps to reduce the number of bacteria on the hands. These should be used when working with high-risk foods. Heavily perfumed soaps should not be used, as they may taint food.

Nails should always be kept short and should be scrubbed whenever the hands are washed because bacteria will collect under them. Nail varnish should not be worn when preparing foods as it easily chips and could fall into food.

Towels rapidly become contaminated with bacteria and an individual method of hand drying is essential. This can either be paper towels together with a foot-operated disposal bin, a linen roller towel or a hot-air drier.

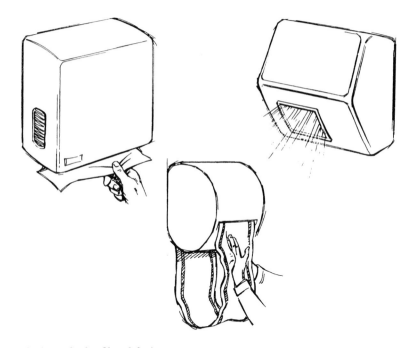

Hygienic methods of hand drying

After thorough drying, hand cream with added disinfectant should be used to keep the skin in good condition. Cracks and grooves in the skin surface or round the nails or knuckles usually harbour Staphylococci bacteria which are not easily removed when the hands are washed.

Hands must always be washed on entering a food room before handling food but even so, unnecessary handling of food should be avoided. Where possible, clean serving tongs should be used, especially for foods which are to be eaten without further cooking, e.g. cream cakes, cooked meats.

**It is very important to wash
the hands after:**

1 ...using the toilet

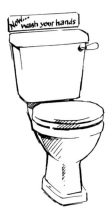

Reason

Bacteria in the faeces can get through toilet paper on to the hands and so on to the food. The faecal–oral route is one of the main ways in which food-borne diseases, such as dysentery, are spread.

2 ...blowing the nose, sneezing or coughing

Approximately 40% of adults harbour Staphylococcus in their nose and throat. Some of these bacteria will be transferred to the hands when a handkerchief is handled. It is preferable to use disposable handkerchiefs which are destroyed after *one* use.

3 ...handling raw meat, poultry or vegetables

The transfer of bacteria from raw meat to cooked dishes (cross-contamination) is a frequent cause of food poisoning. Many raw meat samples have food-poisoning bacteria (usually *C. perfringens* or Salmonella) on the surface. Soil usually contains spores of *C. perfringens*.

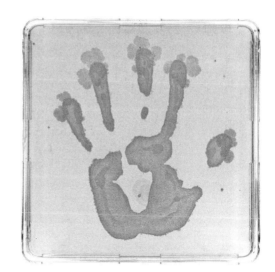

Nutrient agar plate showing the presence of bacteria on the hand after handling raw meat

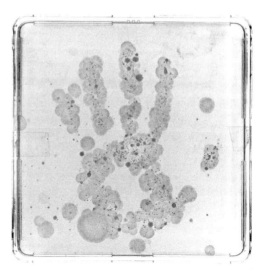

Nutrient agar plate showing the presence of bacteria on the hand after washing vegetables coated with soil

4 ...breaking eggs

Salmonella is often present on eggshells.

5 ...after handling refuse or contaminated food

A great number of all types of bacteria will be present in refuse and waste food.

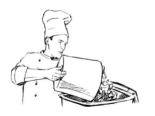

Other aspects of personal and kitchen hygiene

Under no circumstances should food handlers:

1 ...smoke in the kitchen

Reason

It is forbidden by law because bacteria can be transferred from the mouth and lips to the hands. Also, cigarette ends or ash may drop into the food.

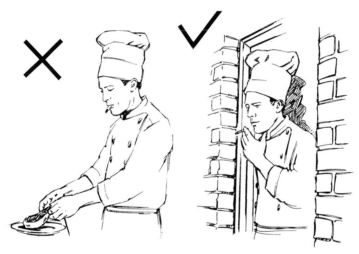

2 ...sneeze or cough over food

Droplets of moisture expelled during coughing and sneezing carry large numbers of Staphylococci bacteria to the food or working surfaces.

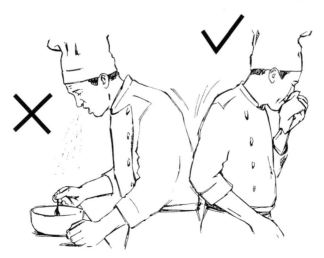

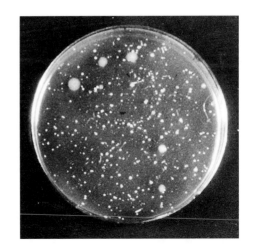

Nutrient agar plate showing bacterial growth produced by a sneeze

3 ...comb their hair in the kitchen Staphylococci bacteria grow well on the scalp and will be transferred to the hands. Loose hairs and dandruff could fall on nearby food. Hair must be washed regularly and covered with a net or hat whilst working in the kitchen.

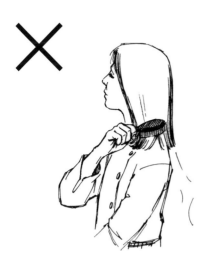

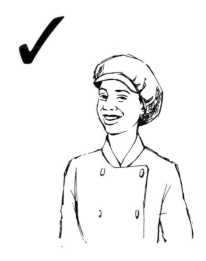

4   …dip their fingers into food to taste it, lick a spoon and return it to the food without washing it or lick their fingers to separate sheets of wrapping paper

Bacteria will be transferred from the mouth to the hands, spoon or paper and so to food.

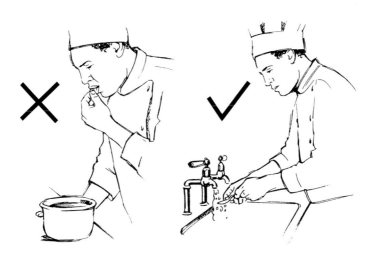

5   …wear any jewellery other than plain wedding rings whilst working in the kitchen

The skin under jewellery tends to harbour a large number of bacteria, especially if the jewellery is not removed in washing. There is always a risk that earrings, tie pins, cufflinks, dress rings, etc. could fall off and become mixed with the food.

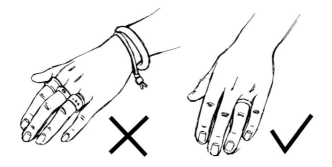

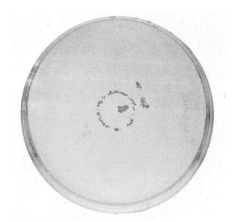

Agar plate showing bacteria present on a ring

It is the duty of every food handler to:

1 …**cover cuts and sores with a coloured waterproof dressing which must be changed regularly. Anyone with a septic cut or a boil, whitlow or stye should stop working with food until medical clearance is given**

Reason

Any cut or sore is likely to be harbouring Staphylococci bacteria. If a coloured dressing accidentally falls off it will be seen before the food is used. If this does happen all the food in the same container must be discarded. It is not satisfactory merely to remove the dressing from the food. Septic cuts, boils, styes and whitlows contain millions of Staphylococci bacteria.

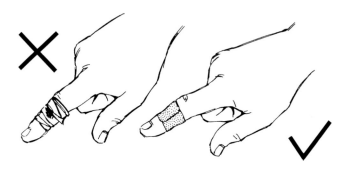

2 …**report any illness, however mild, to his supervisor who will decide whether he is fit to work. This applies particularly to diarrhoea and vomiting, throat and skin infections**

The code of practice *Food Handling – Fitness to Work* provides guidance on how long people should be prevented from working with food after suffering from diarrhoea and vomiting.

Diarrhoea and vomiting are symptoms of food poisoning and even if the condition has cleared up, the employee may still be a convalescent carrier. Staphylococci bacteria are normally present in throat and skin infections.

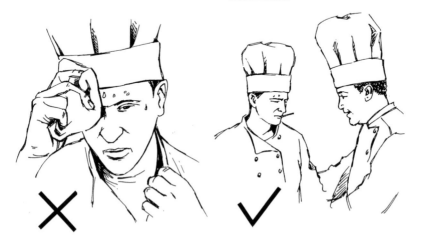

3 ...wear clean overalls, aprons and headgear. Keep sleeves rolled up or securely fastened at the wrists so that cuffs cannot dip into food

Outdoor clothing is frequently contaminated with Staphylococci particularly if it has been worn in congested areas such as on public transport. Clothing lockers should be situated outside the kitchen, making it possible to change into clean, protective clothing before handling food.

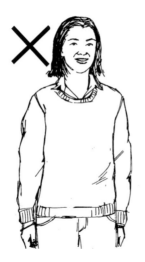
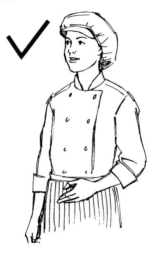

4 ...use clean utensils for food preparation. **Separate work surfaces and chopping boards should be set aside for the preparation of raw meat and must not be used for the preparation of foods which will be eaten without further cooking**

The transfer of bacteria from raw food to cooked food via kitchen utensils or work surfaces is frequently a cause of food poisoning.

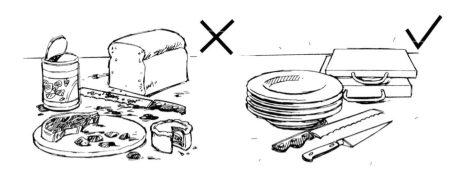

5 ...pick up knives and forks by **their handles, glasses by the stems and plates by the edges**

Bacteria on the hands can be passed to cutlery and crockery and from these articles back to food.

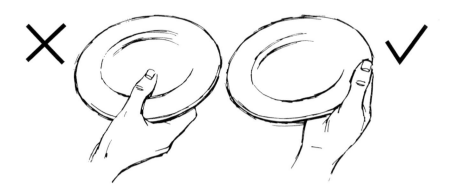

6 ...discard any chipped plates, glasses and damaged utensils

Even an efficient washing-up process may fail to remove bacteria from cracks.

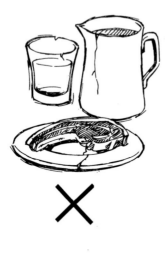

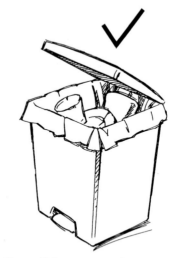

7 ...cover food on display

Flies will be attracted to uncovered food and bacteria in dust particles will settle on the food if it is left uncovered.

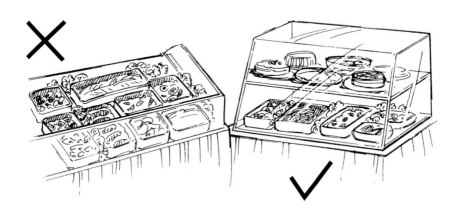

8 ...keep pets out of the kitchen

All animals carry bacteria on their feet and in their fur and these can easily spread into food if the animals are allowed to wander freely in the kitchen.

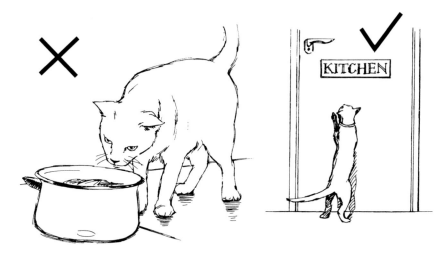

9 ...keep pet food away from human food, using separate utensils for its preparation

Pet food (except canned pet food) is usually heavily contaminated with bacteria.

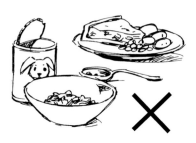
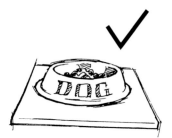

Summary

❑ Maintaining a high standard of personal cleanliness and reporting all illnesses will reduce the risk of causing food poisoning or food-borne diseases.

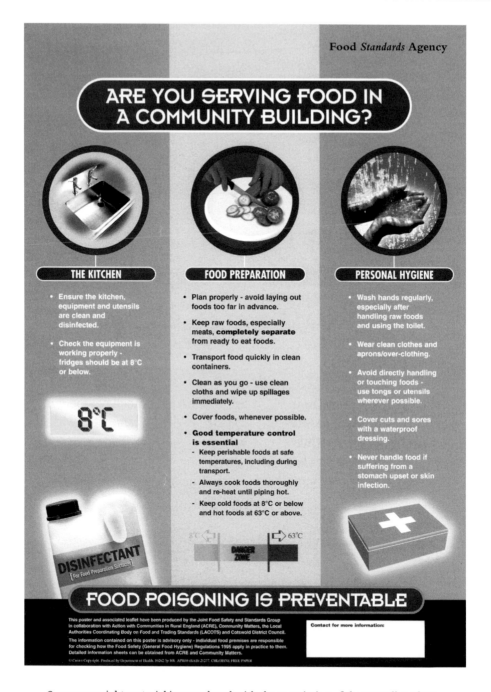

Crown copyright material is reproduced with the permission of the Contoller of Her Majesty's Stationery Office.

14 HYGIENIC FOOD PREPARATION

If the precautions listed in Chapter 13 are observed during food preparation there should be very few harmful bacteria added to the food but further preparation must ensure that those present cannot multiply.

When cooking the food, the combination of cooking time and cooking temperature must be sufficient to destroy bacteria throughout the food. A probe thermometer is very useful for measuring the temperature in the centre of food.

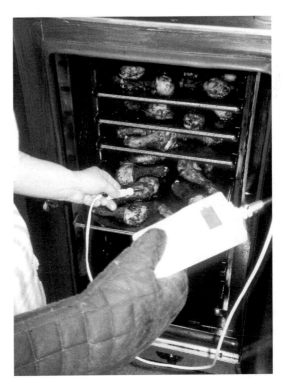

Probe thermometer

Thawing

It is essential that all frozen meats (particularly poultry) should be thawed completely before commencing cooking. If ice is present in the centre of meat it will take far longer for the internal temperature to reach that of the external temperature than in completely defrosted meat. Salmonella food poisoning has frequently been caused because chickens have not been thoroughly defrosted. Although they have been cooked for the recommended time, a great deal of heat is used to melt the remaining ice and the temperature reached in the centre of the bird is not sufficiently high to kill Salmonella but is an optimum temperature for its multiplication.

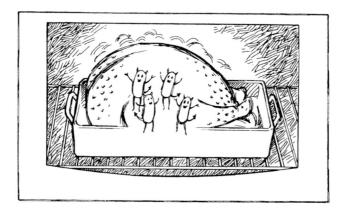

Cooking

Food is a poor conductor of heat and it takes a long time before the temperature in the centre reaches the same temperature as at the surface. For this reason it is safer to reduce the size of rolled joints and minced meats to a maximum of 3 kg (6.6 lb) before cooking them.

Meat and meat products containing raw meat should never be partly cooked one day and the cooking process finished the next day. If the food is only partly cooked it is likely that bacteria will still be alive and even if it is stored in a refrigerator, there will be time for bacteria to multiply during the cooling down process and the second heating process. Just as the centre of joints of meat and meat products only slowly reaches the external temperature when heated up, the temperature at the centre of a hot product drops much more slowly than the temperature at the surface.

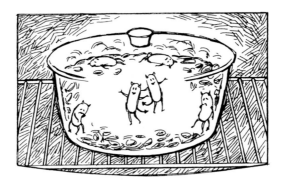

If food has been frozen and thawed it must not be refrozen for the same reason. Bacteria usually remain dormant in frozen food and when the food is thawed they will have a chance to multiply. If the food is then refrozen, a greatly increased number of bacteria will be present, all capable of multiplying next time it is thawed.

Cooling

All foods should be cooled as quickly as possible after cooking so that spore-forming bacteria will have only a short time at a temperature at which they can multiply. Cooked food should not be taken straight from the oven and put into the refrigerator as this will increase the temperature of the refrigerator to a dangerously high level and food-poisoning bacteria may be able to multiply in other foods being stored there.

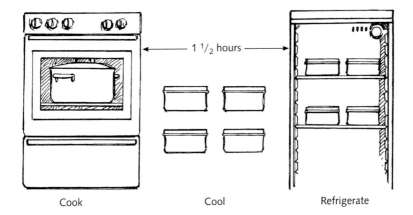

| Cook | Cool | Refrigerate |

Many catering establishments have blast chillers, which are specifically designed to reduce the temperature of the food rapidly before putting it in the refrigerator. If no blast chiller is available, the cooling process can be speeded up by dividing large volumes of hot food into smaller portions. Shallow square or rectangular containers have a greater surface area than deep, circular ones and will allow food to cool more quickly.

Ideally cooked food should be refrigerated within $1\frac{1}{2}$ hours of cooking.

Serving

Any high-risk food must be kept very hot (above 63°C) or very cold (below 5°C). If food is to be eaten hot, it should be served as soon as possible after cooking or kept above 63°C in a holding unit (see p. 94).

If food is to be served cold, it should be stored in a refrigerator until just before it is served.

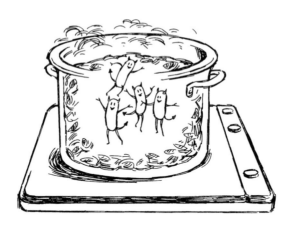

Reheating

Reheating food is always a hazard because cooked food may contain spores of C. perfringens or B. cereus. When the food is cooled the spores will germinate and start to multiply. When the food is reheated, the temperature reached will probably not destroy toxins or spore-forming bacteria.

If reheating is absolutely necessary, the food should be covered and cooled very rapidly after cooking and stored in a refrigerator until it is ready to be reheated. It should then be reheated rapidly and thoroughly. Hot gravy or sauce should never be added to cold food in order to heat it up, since the combined temperature will probably be optimum for bacterial growth.

Meat products and rice should not be reheated more than once because each time a food is reheated there are two opportunities for bacteria to multiply, once during the heating-up process and once during the cooling-down process. In schools and hospitals the usual policy is not to reheat foods at all, since children and sick people are particularly susceptible to food poisoning.

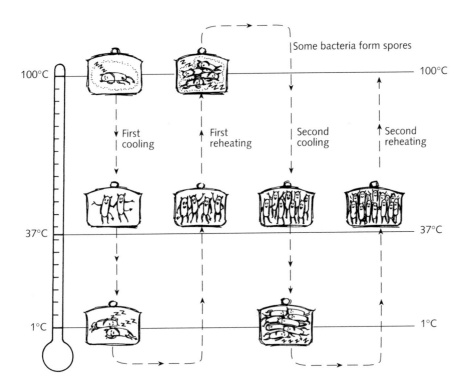

The following table illustrates the fact that food kept at the wrong temperature between preparing and eating, undercooked food, cross-contamination and infected food handlers are the major causes of food poisoning.

FACTORS CONTRIBUTING TO 1426 OUTBREAKS OF FOOD-BORNE INFECTIOUS INTESTINAL DISEASE, ENGLAND AND WALES, 1992–99				
Contributing factor	Salmonella	*C. perfringens*	Other pathogens	Total
Infected food handler	103	2	66	171
Inadequate heat treatment	307	72	61	440
Cross-contamination	295	15	84	394
Storage too long/too warm	259	83	100	442
Other	63	16	50	129
Total	1027	188	361	1576

Source: PHLS GSURV.

Notes: Several factors may contribute to one outbreak.

The outbreak database is now dynamic and therefore the numbers may change slightly over time. However, those quoted are accurate as of 08/03/2001.

Summary

- ❏ All frozen meat should be thoroughly thawed before cooking.
- ❏ Food must be kept either very hot or very cold before it is served and never left at a warm temperature for any length of time.
- ❏ The practice of reheating food should be avoided wherever possible. Meat products and rice must never be reheated more than once.

15 FOODS MOST LIKELY TO CAUSE FOOD POISONING

Some foods favour the growth of food-poisoning bacteria; others do not.

It is not always easy to identify the food which has caused an outbreak as there are frequently no samples of the suspected foods left. However, certain foods are regarded as being 'high risk' and, if eaten just before the illness, will be suspected as the cause. In some of the investigated outbreaks sufficient evidence is available to implicate one particular food.

General outbreaks of Infectious Intestinal Disease, England & Wales, 1992–99

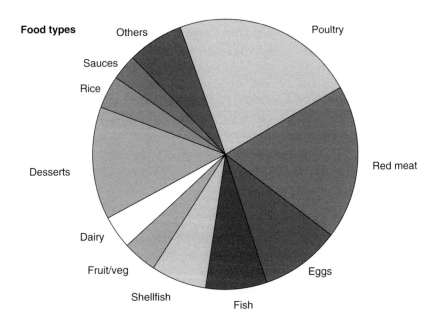

Food types

Others · Poultry · Sauces · Rice · Red meat · Desserts · Dairy · Fruit/veg · Eggs · Shellfish · Fish

Source: PHLS CDSC

High-risk foods

High-risk foods are those that will support bacterial multiplication and will be eaten without further heat treatment. Care must be taken to ensure that they are not contaminated during preparation and are stored correctly prior to service (below 5°C or above 63°C).

Meat and meat products

Every year the majority of food-poisoning outbreaks are caused by meat and meat products.

Freshly roasted meat

Freshly roasted or grilled meat, served hot immediately after cooking, is rarely a cause of food poisoning. As long as a 'rare' steak is cooked on the surface, it will be safe to eat.

Chickens

Most raw chicken carries Salmonella. Freshly roasted chicken (and other poultry) does not normally cause food poisoning unless it has been undercooked. It is advisable to cook stuffing separately, rather than in the cavity of the bird.

Rolled joints

Rolled joints are more frequently a cause of food poisoning because surface meat which may be contaminated will be at the centre of the joint after rolling and also considerable handling by the chef is necessary. It is therefore essential that rolled joints should be small enough to allow sufficient heat to kill bacteria, to penetrate to the centre during cooking.

Cold meats

Cold meats are frequently a cause of food poisoning, usually because they have been contaminated after cooking and kept in a warm environment for several hours before serving.

Stews and casseroles

If served hot immediately after cooking, stews and casseroles will not cause food poisoning. If they are kept warm for several hours or cooled slowly and reheated the next day, there is far more chance that they will cause food poisoning because any spores of *C. perfringens* which survived the first cooking process will have had time to germinate and multiply.

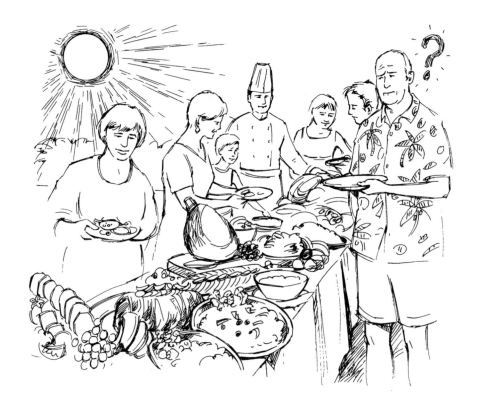

Minced meat
When meat is minced, any pathogenic bacteria which were present on the surface are distributed throughout the mass of the meat.

Beefburgers, pies, pasties, rissoles, sausages and other minced meat dishes
'Made-up' meat dishes are frequently a cause of food poisoning because bacteria may be present throughout the food. Care must be taken to cook the food sufficiently to kill any bacteria in the centre.

Stocks
Stocks and gravies, and soups and sauces made from them are an ideal medium for bacterial growth. They should be kept either hot (above 63°C) until they are served or cold (below 8°C) until they are reheated for service. If they are kept warm for several hours before being reheated for service, they are a likely cause of food poisoning.

Gelatin
Powdered gelatin frequently contains dormant food-poisoning bacteria. When water is added for use in meat pies or as a glaze it becomes an ideal

food for bacterial growth and must therefore be kept at a temperature above 63°C until it is used.

Fish

Freshly cooked fish is rarely a cause of food poisoning because food-poisoning bacteria are not usually present in the intestines of cold-blooded animals. Shellfish sometimes cause food poisoning because they have been gathered from polluted waters. There are, however, strict laws governing the gathering and cleansing of them. Fish dishes such as fish cakes or fish pie may be contaminated during preparation and should therefore always be stored correctly and reheated thoroughly.

Dairy products

Milk

Most milk for sale in the UK has been pasteurised which means that it is free of pathogenic bacteria. However, milk is an ideal food for bacterial growth and could cause food poisoning if contaminated after pasteurisation. Any dishes where milk is an ingredient, such as custards, trifles, milk puddings and sauces, must be served hot or refrigerated until served. Raw (unpasteurised) milk sometimes causes outbreaks of food poisoning or food-borne diseases.

Cream

Cream for sale in most countries has been pasteurised. Cream, like milk, is an ideal food for bacterial growth if it is contaminated after pasteurisation. All cream cakes, trifles, etc. should be kept cold until just before they are served. The same precautions must be taken with imitation cream.

Evaporated and condensed milk

Evaporated milk is safe when the can is first opened but it does support the growth of bacteria. If it is not used straight away, it should be stored in the refrigerator. Condensed milk has a high sugar content, making it unsuitable for bacterial growth.

Dried milk

Dried milk powder contains many dormant bacteria. Once reconstituted, it must be treated as fresh milk and stored in the refrigerator.

Ice cream

Ice cream purchased from a reputable supplier can be regarded as safe. The ingredients will allow bacterial growth and ice cream from an unknown source should not be eaten. Ice cream should not be thawed and then refrozen.

Cheese

In Britain, cheese is normally made from pasteurised milk and is therefore rarely a cause of food poisoning. Hard cheeses do not contain sufficient moisture for bacterial growth but low-fat cheeses do and can be a cause of food poisoning. Soft ripened cheeses such as Brie and Camembert are made from unpasteurised milk and may be contaminated with Listeria (see p. 58).

Eggs

Raw egg is ideal for bacterial growth. Some hens' eggs carry Salmonella inside the shell. It is therefore preferable to cook eggs thoroughly, especially if they are to be eaten by an elderly, very young or sick person, since these people would be more seriously affected by food poisoning. Eggs should be stored in a refrigerator and any cracked eggs should not be used. Pasteurised liquid egg and dried egg are available as safer alternatives to raw egg.

Duck eggs are more frequently contaminated with Salmonella inside the shell and should always be thoroughly cooked.

Egg shells are often contaminated so care must be taken to prevent the transfer of bacteria from the shell to other food in the kitchen.

Rice

Rice is often contaminated with *B. cereus* which forms spores capable of surviving the cooking process. If rice is not eaten immediately after cooking it must be stored in the refrigerator.

Low-risk foods

Certain foods do not normally cause food poisoning because they do not provide bacteria with the nutrients they require for growth and multiplication. Foods with a high concentration of sugar, salt, acid or fat or dry foods will not support the growth of food-poisoning bacteria and are called *low-risk foods*.

Jams, syrup, honey, salted meat

These foods are unlikely to cause food poisoning because the sugar/salt concentration is too high. The sugar and salt present in the food dissolve in the water to form a concentrated solution leaving insufficient moisture for bacterial growth (see Water activity, p. 125).

Fatty foods

Very few types of bacteria can multiply in the presence of high concentrations of fat and those which can are not the ones that cause food poisoning.

Acid foods

Food-poisoning bacteria will not grow in very acid foods such as pickles and citrus fruits (see pH, p. 124).

Dry foods

Dry foods will not support the growth of food-poisoning bacteria but may contain them. If water is added at a later stage in preparation the bacteria will be able to multiply again so the food must then be treated as fresh food and stored in a refrigerator.

Canned foods

In Britain, food is canned and sterilised under strict control and any manufactured canned food can be regarded as safe unless the can is damaged. If it is punctured, has a faulty seam or swollen ends (caused by gas produced inside the can) the manufacturer should be notified and the can and contents either returned or thrown away. Canned ham is often pasteurised only, since sterilisation affects the quality of the ham; it must therefore be stored in a refrigerator. After canned food has been opened it should be handled and stored as fresh food.

Summary

- ❑ Moist, high-protein foods will usually support the growth of food-poisoning bacteria.
- ❑ Foods with a high concentration of sugar, salt, acid or fat or dry foods will not support the growth of food-poisoning bacteria.

16 FOOD STORAGE

Most kitchens have refrigerators, freezers and sometimes cool rooms for low-temperature storage and some means of keeping food very hot when it is about to be served. In addition, microwave ovens are frequently used to reheat foods quickly. The successful use of various combinations of this equipment will ensure that food spends very little time at a temperature within the danger zone.

Deliveries of chilled and frozen food

To ensure that chilled and frozen food is in the best possible condition when it is used, these guidelines should be followed.

❑ Use reputable suppliers, whose delivery vehicles are clean and maintained at the correct temperature.

❑ Reject deliveries of frozen food if it has a temperature above $-10°C$.

❑ Reject deliveries of refrigerated food if it has a temperature above $+10°C$.

❑ Reject frozen food if it shows signs of having been thawed and refrozen, e.g. a solid block of peas.

❑ Check the date coding.

❑ Check the condition of the packaging and reject the food if the packaging is in an unsatisfactory condition. Check for signs of pest damage and mould growth.

Refrigerators

Operating temperature

A refrigerator should operate at a temperature between 1°C and 4°C. Most food-poisoning bacteria will not multiply at this temperature but they will not be killed. During refrigerated storage, food-poisoning bacteria are usually dormant but as soon as the food is removed from the refrigerator and put in a warm room they will start to multiply rapidly. *Clostridium botulinum* and Listeria are exceptions and will multiply slowly at 4°C. Many food spoilage bacteria are able to multiply in the refrigerator but at a much slower rate than at room temperature and so refrigeration only delays spoilage, but will not stop it.

To maintain the correct temperature it is important to:

1   keep the door shut whenever possible

2   cool hot foods before putting them in the refrigerator. Hot foods would cause a considerable increase in the temperature and also condensation which may lead to cross-contamination

3   defrost regularly, unless the refrigerator defrosts automatically. The build-up of excess ice reduces its efficiency and increases the running costs.

The temperature of the refrigerator should not be allowed to drop below 1°C because ice crystals would form in some foods with a high water content, causing loss of texture and quality.

Position of foods

The position of foods in a refrigerator should be carefully planned so that cross-contamination will not occur. Raw meat, poultry, vegetables and fish should be stored separately from prepared food which will not be cooked again. If there is more than one refrigerator in the kitchen, different ones can be used for raw and cooked foods. If there is only one, raw foods should be stored at the bottom of the refrigerator and cooked foods at the top so that contaminated blood or food particles cannot drop from raw food to cooked foods. Strong-smelling foods such as fish should be put in an airtight container and placed as far away as possible from fatty foods which readily absorb smells.

Covering of foods in the refrigerator prevents drying out, cross-contamination and the absorption of odours. Cling film is useful for this purpose but should not be placed over the food until it has cooled. The condensation which

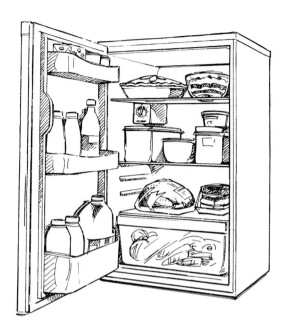

collects when cling film is placed over warm food speeds up spoilage of that food. Cling film should not be allowed to touch the food it is covering and so should not be used to wrap foods, particularly those which have a high fat content, e.g. cheese. The 'clinging' properties of cling film come from substances known as plasticisers present in the film. These plasticisers have been shown to migrate into fatty foods when the film is in direct contact with the food. The migration of plasticisers increases when the cling film is heated and for this reason it should not be used in contact with food in a microwave or conventional oven.

A refrigerator functions by circulating cold air round the food so it is essential that it is not so tightly packed that the circulation of air is restricted.

Commercial refrigeration units

There are many designs of refrigeration units for use in large catering establishments. The basic unit is the 'reach-in' cabinet which is available in many sizes. Any combination of removable internal fittings such as shelves or deep containers can be chosen depending on storage requirements. All these are removable to facilitate cleaning. Stainless steel doors are usually fitted to withstand tough treatment in busy kitchens.

For even larger quantities, 'roll-in' refrigerators are available which will accommodate trolleys of food. Some have a door at the preparation end and a door at the opposite end which opens in the serving area.

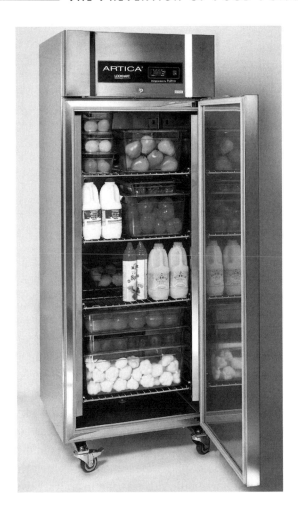

Other refrigeration units include mobile refrigerators for food which is to be served a distance from the preparation area and refrigerators with glass doors which can be used for displaying food such as cream cakes and other desserts or for cold drinks and wine. Refrigerators with glass doors must not be positioned so that the door is in direct sunlight because this allows heat to build up in the refrigerator in the same way as it does in a greenhouse.

In all commercial premises, refrigerator temperature checks should be made three times each day and the results recorded. If the temperature varies much from the ideal temperature, action must be taken.

Regular cleaning and disinfection should also take place, particularly of the internal surfaces and the door handles. A cleaning schedule should be devised and a record made of each cleaning operation.

Chillers

A refrigerator should not be used to cool hot food and in a catering establishment where large volumes of food such as roast meats and poultry must be cooled quickly before refrigerating, a blast chiller is almost essential. The temperature of the food is reduced quickly to 15°C due to the circulation of a continuous current of cold air.

Freezers

Operating temperature

The length of time for which food can be safely stored in a freezer depends on the temperature of the freezer. Most domestic freezers operate at -18°C and are capable of freezing fresh food without affecting the temperature of the frozen food already in the cabinet. Some bacteria will be killed during storage at this temperature but many can remain dormant for long periods of time. Spores and toxins are not affected by freezing. When food is taken out of the freezer and thawed, the surviving bacteria start to grow and multiply again. Food that has been frozen tends to allow more rapid bacterial growth than the equivalent fresh food and therefore deteriorates rather more quickly.

Defrosting

Some foods can be cooked straight from the freezer but joints and larger volumes of meat must be completely defrosted before cooking.

Ideally, food should be defrosted in a thawing cabinet at a temperature between 10°C and 15°C.

Defrosting in a refrigerator is slow (about four days for a large turkey) and there is a substantial risk of cross-contaminating other foods and the surfaces of the refrigerator with the thawed liquid.

Defrosting at room temperature will allow spoilage and pathogenic bacteria to grow on the surface while the centre is still defrosting.

The thawing cabinet must be cleaned and disinfected regularly. It must not be used for storage of food.

Refreezing

Food should not be refrozen once it has thawed unless it is cooked in between. There are two reasons for this.

1 If the thawed food is kept at room temperature for some time, any pathogenic bacteria present will have a chance to multiply.

2 The texture of the food will suffer. Large ice crystals tend to form when food is frozen relatively slowly in domestic freezers. The loss of texture which this causes is more noticeable in food which has been thawed and refrozen.

Freezer breakdown

If there is a power cut or the freezer breaks down, the door or lid should be kept closed and covered with blankets to minimise the temperature increase. If the food is still frozen when the power is restored or the freezer is mended, it may be safe to keep the food. If in doubt, an environmental health officer will give advice on this matter. If the food has thawed out, one of the following options must be chosen.

1 Use the food immediately.

2 Store the food in a refrigerator but for no longer than two days.

3 Cook the food thoroughly, cool rapidly and freeze or store in a refrigerator for no longer than three days.

4 Destroy the food.

Food stores

Dried foods, canned and bottled foods and fruit and vegetables should ideally be kept in a well-ventilated store, which maintains a temperature between 10°C and 15°C.

Goods should be stored away from the walls and above floor level and the store must be well lit to aid cleaning and the detection of pests.

Microwave ovens

Microwave ovens provide a quick and convenient way of cooking and reheating food provided they are used correctly.

Any catering establishment that uses a microwave oven regularly for cooking or reheating should use a commercial model. Domestic microwave ovens have a life expectancy of 2000 hours and an output of between 500 and 700 watts, whereas commercial microwave ovens are designed to last for many more hours of use and have an output of between 700 and 1600 watts. Food can therefore be defrosted, cooked and reheated more efficiently in a commercial microwave oven.

In order to ensure that food cooked in a microwave oven does not cause food poisoning, the same principles that apply in conventional cooking must be followed.

1   Defrost food completely before starting to cook it.

2   Cook food thoroughly, by cooking it for the required length of time on the correct power setting. The temperature in the centre of the food should reach 82°C. The time required to reach this temperature will depend on the density and quantity of the food.

3   Observe standing times, as this is part of the cooking process.

4   Never reheat meat or rice, or foods containing them, more than once.

It can be useful to make a table similar to the one below, which gives the correct cooking times and standing times, for the foods most frequently handled.

Food	Setting	Time	Standing time
Trout (6 oz)	Defrost	$2\frac{1}{2}$ min	1 min
Chicken joint (8 oz)	Defrost	3 min	2 min
Plated meal (16 oz)	Defrost	$5\frac{1}{2}$ min	2 min
Frozen sandwich	Defrost	$1\frac{1}{2}$ min	30 sec
Meat pie (5 oz)	Heating	25 sec	30 sec
Meat pie (5 oz) × 5	Heating	$1\frac{1}{4}$ min	1 min
Plated meal (16 oz)	Heating	$1\frac{1}{2}$ min	1 min
Apple pie – 8 portions	Heating	$3\frac{1}{2}$ min	1 min
Pizza (8 in)	Heating	40 sec	30 sec
Pizza (8 in) × 4	Heating	60 sec	1 min
Chicken (3 lb 6 oz)	Cooking	16 min	3 min
Trout (6 oz)	Cooking	1 min	30 sec
Frozen peas (2 lb)	Cooking	$4\frac{1}{2}$ min	–

Microwave ovens should be cleaned regularly, in particular around the door seal because the presence of dirt and grease may stop the door closing correctly. They should be checked every year to ensure there is no leakage of microwaves. Local environmental health departments often provide a testing service.

Holding units

Many kitchens have a hot cupboard and/or a bain-marie for keeping food warm for short periods of time just before it is served. A hot cupboard is heated by gas or electricity and a bain-marie is a heated well filled with hot water. Both systems should be hot enough to ensure that the temperature at the centre of the food is kept above 63°C. They must never be used for heating up cold foods as the process would be too slow using either piece of equipment.

Cook-chill and cook-freeze systems

These methods of food preparation are becoming increasingly common and are widely used in situations where a large number of meals have to be served a long distance from the kitchens where they are prepared, such as aeroplanes, and some hospitals and schools. In any of these situations it would be unsatisfactory to cook the food and keep it warm until it is required. In cook-chill and cook-freeze systems the food is prepared in the central preparation unit: it is cooked thoroughly and then divided into individual portions observing strict hygiene standards. All containers are marked with the date (to ensure effective stock rotation) and also with the contents, reheating time and any other instructions.

Cook-chill

The food is chilled in a blast chiller to between 1°C and 3°C within two hours of cooking and must be kept in a refrigerator at this temperature until it is required for distribution. It should be reheated within two hours of arrival at the point of consumption. The temperature in the centre of the food should reach 82°C and must be held at 63°C or above until it is served. All meals must be eaten within five days including the day of preparation.

A bacterium called *Listeria monocytogenes* grows slowly at refrigeration temperatures. It is therefore important to observe the storage instructions, the 'eat by' date on the cover and the heating instructions. The bacterium does not form a spore and thorough heating of the meal will make it safe to eat. Great care must be taken to ensure thorough and uniform heating if cook-chill meals are reheated in a microwave. The food must be cooked for the required length of time on the stated power setting and in the correct position. Instructions for standing times must also be observed because the food is continuing to cook by conduction during this period.

Cook-freeze

The food is blast frozen (a very rapid method of freezing) to a temperature of $-20°C$ within $1\frac{1}{2}$ hours and kept at this temperature for up to 12 months. When it is reheated, the temperature in the centre of the food should reach 82°C and must be held at 63°C or above until it is served.

Whichever system is used, any reheated food which is not consumed must be discarded.

It is important to bear in mind that any departure from these guidelines could result in an outbreak of food poisoning involving a large number of people. Further details can be obtained from the DoH code of practice *Guidelines on Precooked Chilled Foods*.

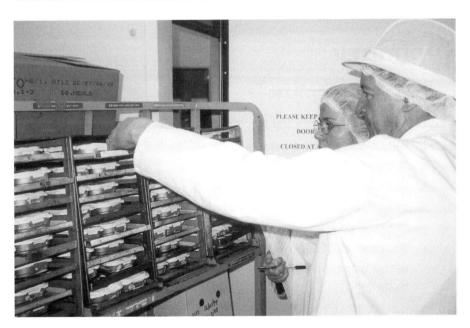

Date marking

Food-labelling regulations introduced in January 1991 made it compulsory for most foods to carry a date mark. The date mark on a food is the date before which the food should be eaten. If the food has been stored correctly it will be fresh and safe to eat on this date but the quality cannot be guaranteed beyond it.

The date mark can be in one of three forms.

1   For foods that keep for three months or less
    'BEST BEFORE' followed by the day and month.

2   For foods that keep for more than 3 months
    'BEST BEFORE END' followed by the month and year.

3   For highly perishable foods, that is, those likely to cause illness if not eaten in the recommended time
    'USE BY' followed by the day and month.

It is an offence to sell food for consumption after the 'use by' date.

Any special storage conditions necessary should appear after each date mark, e.g. 'store in a refrigerator'.

Summary

- ❏   The temperature of a refrigerator must be maintained between 1°C and 4°C.
- ❏   Frozen food should not be refrozen once it has thawed.
- ❏   Microwave ovens provide a quick method of cooking and reheating food.
- ❏   Holding units must be hot enough to maintain a food temperature of 63°C or above. They must not be used for heating up cold foods.
- ❏   The cook-chill and cook-freeze methods of food preparation are useful when food has to be cooked some distance from where it is to be served.

17 CLEANING AND DISINFECTION

High standards of cleanliness in food premises are a legal requirement but they will also create a pleasant working environment and promote a favourable image to potential customers.

Cleaning removes grease and dirt. Hot water and detergent are normally used to clean kitchen equipment.

Disinfection removes vegetative bacteria, but not spores. Disinfection can be achieved by the use of very hot water on its own or by the use of chemicals.

Sterilisation removes all bacteria and their spores. Sterilisation can be achieved by the use of steam or chemicals. It is not necessary to sterilise equipment used for food preparation: disinfecting it is adequate.

Detergents

Detergents are chemicals which, when added to water, help to remove grease, dirt and food residues.

A detergent does not kill bacteria but reduces the number present on an article by removing the dirt and grease that harbour them. If water without detergent is used on a greasy surface, the water tends to form droplets and will not remove the food residues effectively. Detergents are most effective when used with hot water.

Stage I

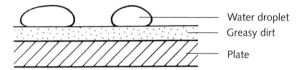

Water does not spread evenly on greasy plates and tends to form small droplets

Stage II

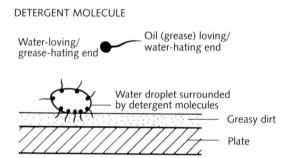

Detergent is added to the water;
The detergent molecules surround the water droplets;
The head of the molecule (water-loving end) enters the water;
The tail (water-hating end) is attracted to the grease.

Stage III

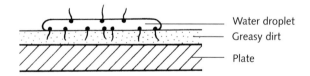

The water now spreads on the grease;
The detergent molecules 'fasten' the water and grease together;
Rubbing with a cloth or sponge removes grease and dirt together from the plate.

Stage IV

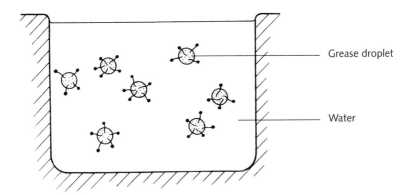

The grease now rolls up into drops surrounded by detergent molecules and is suspended in the water. When the water goes down the drain the grease goes with it.

Washing-up liquid is a detergent used in the home and in industrial kitchens to clean utensils and most equipment. Its action is fairly mild and other detergents are available for heavily soiled equipment. A very alkaline detergent is used in dishwashers and can be used for removing baked-on grease from kitchen equipment.

Disinfectants

The best method of disinfecting kitchen equipment is to immerse it in very hot water (80–88°C) for two to three minutes. This method should be used whenever possible but if it is not practicable a chemical disinfectant can be used. The ones most commonly used in catering premises contain either hypochlorites or iodophors as the active ingredient.

Hypochlorites are inexpensive and provided they are used at the correct dilution, are very effective and leave little taste or smell. For disinfection they must be left in contact with the equipment for a specific time, called the 'contact time'. The main disadvantage of hypochlorites is that they are easily inactivated by food particles and so are only effective when the equipment has already been thoroughly cleaned with hot water and a detergent. If hypochlorites are mixed with some types of acid cleaning agents, they can release chorine gas, which is harmful. The manufacturer's instructions must be followed carefully to ensure that the correct combination of cleaning agents is used in the correct concentrations.

Iodophors disinfect surfaces rapidly, leaving little taste and smell, but again are easily inactivated by food residues. Cleaning materials containing iodophors tend to be more expensive than those containing hypochlorites.

When to disinfect

Some surfaces and equipment in a kitchen do not need to be disinfected. For example, a detergent wash is sufficient for floors and walls.

Disinfection after cleaning is normally considered necessary for:

❑　kitchen equipment in direct contact with food, e.g. chopping boards, work surfaces, knives and other utensils, mixing bowls

❑　equipment touched by the food handler during preparation, e.g. refrigerator door handles, taps, oven doors

❑　cleaning equipment, e.g. cloths, brushes and mops. Colour coding of cleaning equipment is also advisable to ensure that the same equipment is not used in raw food preparation areas and high-risk areas

❑　the hands of a food handler. Frequent washing in hot, soapy water is normally considered adequate. When handling high-risk foods, it is preferable to apply a disinfectant after hand washing.

Sanitisers (also called bactericidal detergents)

Sanitisers are chemicals which combine both a detergent and disinfectant. Chemical disinfectants are partially inactivated by dirt and food residues, so sanitisers are not as effective for dirty equipment and surfaces as a detergent wash followed by disinfection. They are suitable for lightly soiled equipment or surfaces.

Cleaning and disinfection procedures

There are six basic stages in any cleaning and disinfection process, whether it is for cleaning large equipment, cleaning work surfaces or washing up. In some cleaning processes, two or more of the following stages may be combined.

1   *Pre-clean* – removal of loose dirt and food residues by scraping or wiping. This stage may include soaking or rinsing.

2   *Main clean* – loosening and removing the remaining dirt and food residues by using a detergent and a cleaning cloth, brush or jet of water.

3   *Intermediate rinse* – removal of any remaining dirt and any detergent.

4   *Disinfection* – destruction of bacteria to a level appropriate for food use.

5   *Final rinse* – removal of chemical disinfectant, if it has been used.

6   *Drying* – preferably air drying or by the use of a dry, clean tea towel or disposable paper towels.

Washing-up procedure

In a commercial kitchen washing up should not take place in a food preparation area because of the danger of dirty plates contaminating work surfaces which are to be used for the preparation of food. If a kitchen serves a canteen or restaurant, the washing-up area should be next to the exit door from the restaurant so that dirty crockery and utensils need not be brought into the food preparation area at all. Washing up can be done either by hand, in which case at least two sinks are necessary, or by a dish-washing machine. Whichever method is used, the process is similar.

1   *Preparation* – crockery should be scraped clean and if possible all crockery and utensils should be given a pre-rinse in warm water so that the washing water at the next stage will stay cleaner.

2   *Main wash* – at this stage a detergent is added to the water to help remove food remains and grease.

    The temperature of the water should be between 50°C and 60°C. This is too hot for bare hands so rubber gloves will be needed. It should not exceed 63°C because certain protein residues such as traces of egg become baked on to plates and cutlery if water hotter than this is used. Wiping with a clean nylon brush or a disposable dishcloth in this combination of hot water and detergent will remove grease and food residues but it will not make the equipment completely free from bacteria.

    The washing-up water must be changed frequently and more detergent added so it will always be both clean and at the correct temperature.

3   *Rinsing stage* – the articles are transferred from the sink which contains water and detergent into a sink containing very hot water at a

temperature of about 80°C. They are left immersed in the water for 2 minutes. The purpose of this stage is:

❏ to rinse off any traces of detergent

❏ to kill any remaining bacteria

❏ to heat the articles to a sufficiently high temperature to allow them to air dry.

4   *Drying* – it is generally considered best to allow crockery and utensils to drain dry in racks. They will dry fairly quickly if the temperature of the rinse water is maintained at 80°C. Clean, dry crockery and utensils should be stored under cover so that they will not be recontaminated.

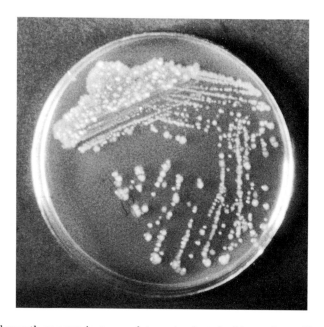

Bacterial growth on a nutrient agar plate contaminated with one drop of liquid from a dirty dishcloth

Guidelines for the use of cleaning chemicals

1   Store chemicals away from food, preferably in a cool, dry storeroom.

2   Store chemical containers in an upright position and firmly closed.

3   Ensure all containers are labelled correctly. Never use empty food or drink containers for storing chemicals because of the risk of a mistake being made.

4   Follow the manufacturer's instructions about dilution rates. A solution that is too strong may damage surfaces, one that is too weak will be ineffective.

5   Make a fresh solution at least daily.

6   Do not leave cloths, mops or brushes in a disinfectant solution which has been used. The dirt will inactivate the disinfectant and the cleaning equipment will become a breeding ground for micro-organisms.

Dish-washing machines

There are many different types of dish-washing machines all of which vary slightly in their operation. It is therefore important to follow the manufacturer's instructions. The principle is the same as for the hand-washing method. Dirty crockery and utensils are stacked into the machine, pre-rinsed, washed in water at 60°C and a detergent, and then rinsed at a temperature between 80°C and 88°C. They should be allowed to air-dry under cover.

It is essential that regular checks are made to ensure that the dish-washing machine is working correctly. Most industrial machines have dials on the outside so that the operator can check that the temperatures of the water are correct and that the articles are exposed to the very hot rinsing water for the correct length of time.

Glassware

Glassware should be washed in a machine or by a two-sink method with detergent and water at 50–60°C in the first sink and water at 80°C in the second sink. If the glassware will not stand this temperature, a chemical disinfectant must be added to the second sink. Small glass-washing machines which can be fixed to the bar itself are often used in licensed premises. A sanitiser is added to the water and the cleaning action is performed by revolving brushes whilst the glass is held in place by hand. Machines with a separate rinsing chamber are preferable to single-chamber machines.

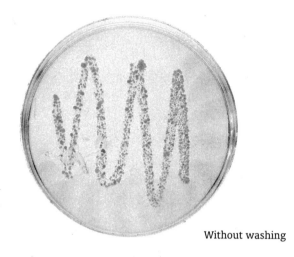

Without washing

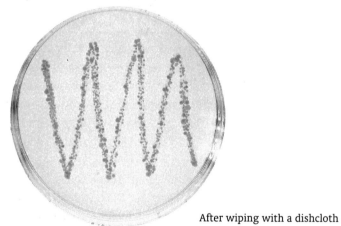

After wiping with a dishcloth

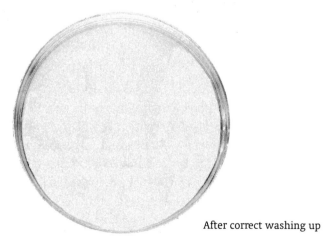

After correct washing up

Nutrient agar plates showing bacteria present on a chopping board after preparing raw meat

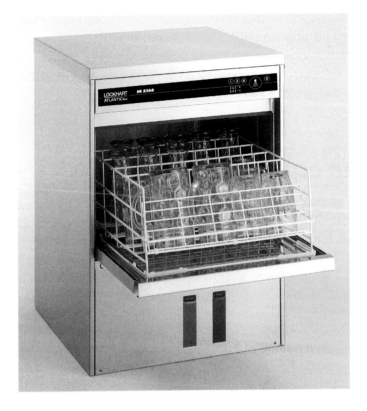

Glass-washing machine

Washing pans

Pots, pans and other cooking vessels should be washed separately from crockery and cutlery. A tap proportioner can be fitted which will draw the correct amount of detergent from a container and mix it with the water. Scouring pads should be available. Stubborn grease can be removed by adding an alkali such as washing soda (sodium bicarbonate).

Working surfaces

Working surfaces should be cleaned as follows.

1   Wipe off crumbs and loose dirt.

2   Wash down with a detergent and water at a temperature of 50–60°C using a disposable cloth.

3   Rinse thoroughly with a chemical disinfectant added to the water. This disinfectant solution must remain in contact with the surface for the time recommended in the instructions. Sanitisers (a detergent combined with a disinfectant) can be used for surfaces that are visibly clean, in which case stages 2 and 3 are combined.

Other equipment

A cleaning routine should be established for all articles of equipment in use in the kitchen. As a general rule, all equipment which comes into direct contact with food should be cleaned after every use. Other surfaces and equipment should be cleaned as necessary. To ensure that cleaning is not overlooked it is a good idea to draw up a cleaning schedule which lists the items to be cleaned, the frequency and method of cleaning and the name of the person to whom the task is allotted.

The person responsible should sign on completion of the task and a supervisor should sign when they have checked that the cleaning task has been satisfactorily completed. It may be necessary to swab surfaces to ensure that cleaning methods are satisfactory. Rapid bacterial testing swabs are available for this purpose.

Item	Frequency	Allocated to:	Date completed:	Checked by:
Bins and refuse areas	Daily			
Floors	Twice daily			
Walls	Weekly			
Freezer	Every two weeks			

Dish washing at home

If a dishwasher is not available, the temperatures used for washing with detergent and for rinsing should be the same as in commercial premises. Rubber gloves will therefore be needed.

It is important to remember that clean crockery and utensils can easily be recontaminated by a dirty tea towel. If tea towels are used for drying, they should be washed after each use. If the crockery and utensils are left to dry in the air they should be stacked away under cover as soon as they are dry and before preparation and cooking of food begins again.

Summary

❏ Detergents remove dirt and grease but do not kill bacteria.

❏ Disinfectants kill the majority of bacteria on surfaces and equipment.

❏ Washing up can be done by hand or machine. In both cases the articles to be cleaned are subjected to a detergent wash and are then rinsed in water that is hot enough to disinfect.

❏ Surfaces and equipment in contact with food should be cleaned and disinfected after use.

❏ Cleaning equipment must be cleaned and disinfected after use.

❏ A cleaning schedule must be established for large equipment and premises.

18 KITCHEN DESIGN

It would be unrealistic for anyone to think that a kitchen can be made free from bacteria but there are several general principles concerning kitchen design and the layout of equipment which will help to reduce the risk of cross-contamination of foods.

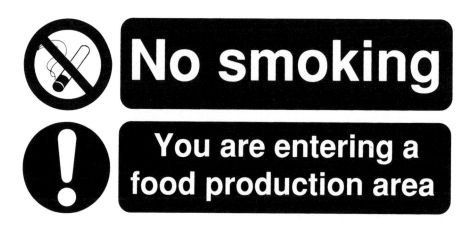

The main consideration in designing a kitchen is that the layout should allow easy cleaning and a continuous workflow from receiving raw foods through preparation and cooking to final presentation. Equipment should be movable or should be placed where it is possible to clean at the back, sides and underneath as well as at the front. If the equipment is not movable, it should, where possible, be built in with one continuous surface between the equipment and the wall or floor so that dirt and grease cannot lodge in joints and corners.

A spacious kitchen is easier to keep clean and run hygienically than a small cramped kitchen. In a kitchen serving a restaurant, there must always be a division of preparation areas bearing the following points in mind.

1   Vegetable storage and preparation should be near to the delivery door. Potatoes and other vegetables have soil on them which carries *C. perfringens* spores and if the vegetables are carried through the kitchen, dust from the vegetables may easily settle on cooked food.

2   Sections for raw meat preparation and cooked food preparation should be well separated to avoid cross-contamination because raw meat is frequently contaminated with Salmonella and *C. perfringens* bacteria.

Food preparation area
Cooked food only

Pastry
preparation area

3   The washing-up area should not be near the preparation areas so that dirty crockery and food waste will not come into contact with food to be eaten.

Plan for a restaurant kitchen

The layout will vary, depending on the size and shape of the premises and the food being prepared, but the main aim is to have a continuous work flow, which keeps clean and dirty processes well separated. These principles are illustrated by the design shown in the illustration opposite.

Lighting

In all kitchens it is essential that there is adequate lighting.

Natural light puts less strain on the eyes than artificial light so windows should be large. Artificial light will of course be needed at times and should be bright enough to prevent accidents happening during food preparation and should be shadow-free so that all dirt is readily visible and the kitchen can be cleaned properly.

Ventilation

Adequate ventilation in a kitchen is very important for two reasons.

1　To keep the temperature and humidity down. (The temperature and humidity of a hot steamy kitchen are ideal for bacterial growth.)

2　To remove cooking smells, steam, grease, etc.

In a large industrial kitchen, hoods connected to extractor fans are usually fitted over the cookers. These must be cleaned regularly because grease and dirt reduce their efficiency.

Windows which are opened for ventilation should be screened to prevent entry of insects and birds.

Working surfaces

Working surfaces should be made from a hard-wearing easily cleaned material which will not absorb moisture, chip or crack, and will not be affected by food residues. Stainless steel is the usual choice but food-grade plastic laminates may also be suitable, providing the gaps between the sheets are sealed. Gaps and cracks will harbour food residues and hence

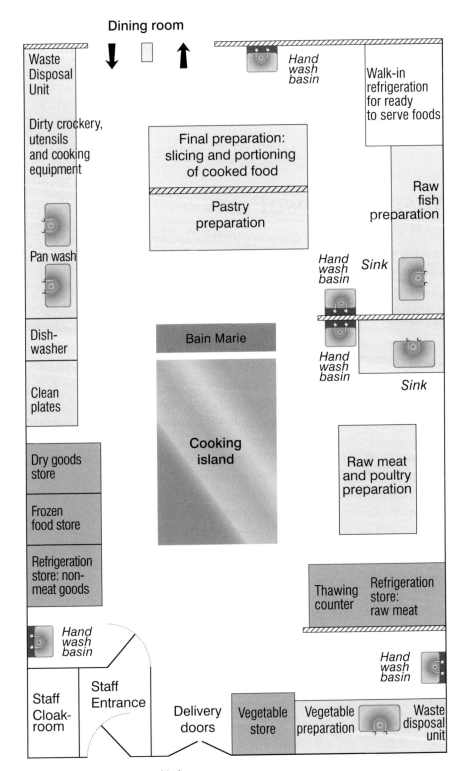

A well-planned restaurant kitchen

bacteria. Wooden working surfaces should not be used as these rapidly become contaminated and are difficult to clean. Hardwood is still used for chopping boards but laminated plastic boards are preferable, because they can be washed in a dishwasher.

Wood boards are sometimes still used for raw meat but they should be kept for that purpose only. Colour coding the board red will remind staff of this (see p. 22).

Waste disposal

Food waste is ideal for the growth of bacteria and unless it is carefully protected it will attract flies, rats, mice and other pests which may then transfer the bacteria back to fresh food in the kitchen.

Left-over food and residues from food preparation should be removed from the working area immediately and put into pedal bins lined with plastic sacks. Disposable paper sacks with pedal-operated metal lids can be used for dry waste. There should be an adequate number of bins in the kitchen so that waste does not have to be carried across the kitchen. The bins must never be allowed to overflow and should be emptied regularly at the end of the day, even if not full, in order to remove a source of food for pests. It is essential to wash the hands after handling refuse and before handling food again.

A special area outside and not too near the kitchen window should be set aside for bins containing refuse and awaiting disposal. They should have tight-fitting lids so that they cannot be knocked off by animals or blown off by the wind. An uncovered dustbin will attract flies and other pests. The bins

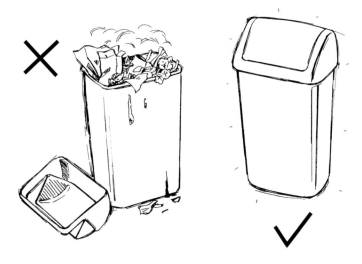

should have rounded comers to facilitate cleaning and be placed on a metal stand approximately one foot above a drained and concreted area which should be washed down frequently. Alternatively, large heavy-duty wheeled bins can be used.

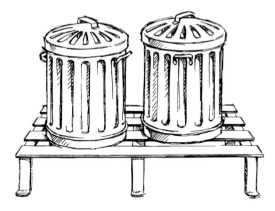

Dustbins – correct type and storage

Waste disposal units

These are a modern and convenient way of dealing with waste. They are made up of a system of high-speed cutters which shred the waste food which is then washed away into the drainage system.

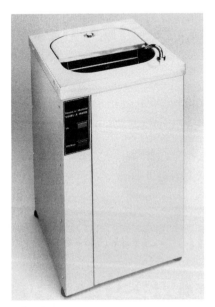

Food waste disposal unit

Washing facilities

An adequate number of hand-washing basins with hot and cold water, soap, a nailbrush and drying facilities must be present in convenient positions, e.g. at the entrance to the kitchen and next to the preparation areas. These must not be used for food preparation.

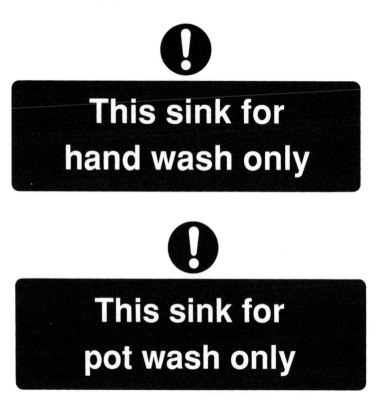

Stainless steel sinks should be located in each preparation area for washing food and must not be used for washing hands.

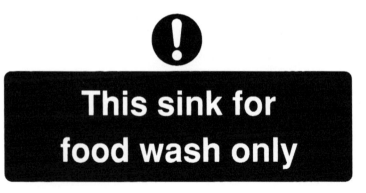

Floors

Kitchen floors should be made of a hard-wearing, anti-slip, easily cleaned material which will not absorb moisture and will not be affected by food residues such as grease, salt and fruit acids. Non-slip quarry tiles laid in acid-resisting cement and thick, non-slip vinyl sheets are both suitable. There should be no breaks or cracks in the surface as these will allow dirt and bacteria to accumulate. The junction of the floor with the wall should be coved (rounded).

Ceilings

Ceilings should have a smooth finish to facilitate cleaning. Stove-enamelled metal tiles or plasterboard sheeting coved to the wall is suitable. Polystyrene tiles are unsuitable because of the fire risk and because they are difficult to clean.

Walls

Walls should have smooth surfaces which will be easy to clean and should be light-coloured to make dirt easily visible. Areas which frequently become soiled, e.g. around sinks and cooking apparatus, are best covered with either stainless steel sheets or ceramic tiles. Areas less susceptible to splashing (above 1.5 m/5 ft) can be painted with a steam-resistant emulsion.

Summary

- A well-planned, easily cleaned kitchen will save time and effort in food preparation and will reduce the risk of contamination of food.
- The kitchen must be well lit and ventilated.
- Floors, walls and working surfaces should be made from smooth hard-wearing and non-absorbent materials.
- An adequate number of hand-washing basins and food preparation sinks must be present.
- Waste disposal units or disposable plastic or paper sacks which are removed from the kitchen regularly are the most hygienic methods of waste disposal.

19 KITCHEN PESTS

Rats, mice, flies and cockroaches are the most common kitchen pests. Clean, well-constructed and well-maintained premises will not harbour any of these pests and it is therefore the duty of the food handler to make the premises where he works unattractive to pests by maintaining a high standard of hygiene and by keeping buildings in good repair.

Rats and mice

The brown rat and the house mouse are the most common rodent pests found in kitchens. They live and breed in warm dark corners where they will not be disturbed and where food is plentiful and easily accessible. In one year about 200 rats can be produced from one pair of rats and their young and one pair of mice and their young can produce up to 2000 offspring.

Rats and mice prefer cereals but will eat almost any food which is easily accessible to them.

The main problem is not the quantity of food pests eat but the amount they contaminate with harmful bacteria. Rats and mice frequently carry Salmonella in their intestines and so their droppings will contain live bacteria. They also carry bacteria on their fur and feet and can therefore transfer food-poisoning bacteria from soil, waste food and refuse to uncovered food and surfaces used for food preparation just by running over them.

The bacterium which causes Weil's disease can be present in a rat's urine. Weil's disease causes jaundice and can be fatal.

Rats and mice need to wear down their incisor teeth which grow continuously. They do this by gnawing woodwork, water pipes and electrical cables. They have been known to cause fires and floods and often make costly repairs necessary.

Signs of a rodent infestation

❏ Droppings

❏ Paw marks in dust, flour and grain

❏ Torn packets

❏ Gnawing marks

❏ Greasy marks on paintwork from the rat's fur and tail.

Preventing a rodent infestation

❏ Keep food premises in good repair.

❏ Block up holes in the building apart from air bricks which should have a wire mesh behind them.

❏ Ensure the doors fit well and are kept closed when not in use. Wooden doors should have metal plates on the bottom of them.

❏ Check there is no access for pests via false ceilings or boxed-in pipe work. Pipe runs should be sealed at the entrance to the building and where they pass from room to room.

❏ Bins must have well-fitting lids and be emptied regularly.

❏ Clean up any spillages.

❏ Repair dripping taps and any leaks in the roof to deny pests water.

❏ Check all deliveries on arrival to ensure they are free of pests.

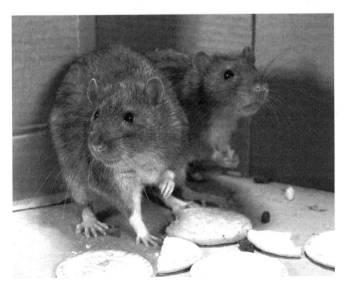

Brown rats

Treating an infestation

In the event of an infestation of rats or mice expert advice should be sought. A local authority environmental health department will offer advice and possibly a treatment. Alternatively a reputable pest control contractor (preferably a member of the British Pest Control Association) should be employed. He will survey the premises, suggest any improvements which should be made and detect, monitor and treat pests as necessary on an agreed contract basis.

Rats and mice are usually eliminated with poisons (rodenticides) which are laid in tamper-resistant bait boxes, as a solid block or in a paste formulation. These methods aim to reduce the risk of contamination of food with rodenticide. Rats are very suspicious animals and may not take the bait in the first few days.

Traps or sticky boards can be used for the occasional invader but would not be suitable in the case of a large infestation. The advantage of traps is that the rodent's body can be removed and disposed of safely whereas with chemical methods the rodent can hide and die somewhere inaccessible such as under the floorboards. This may cause a smell from the decomposing body.

Houseflies and bluebottles

The number of flies in an urban environment has decreased significantly due to more efficient disposal of refuse and sewage but the fly is still a common pest in summer months. It feeds on refuse, from which it flies to human food where it deposits bacteria from its legs, wings, saliva and excrement.

Flies breed very rapidly. They lay their eggs in warm, moist places such as on waste food and refuse. At summer temperatures it takes only ten days for the egg to develop into a maggot and then into an adult fly.

Bluebottles are characterised by their large size, their blue colour and the buzzing noise they make whilst flying. They are attracted to meat and fish products on which they lay their eggs.

The most effective method of reducing the number of flies in a kitchen is to cover windows, door spaces and ventilators with a gauze which is too fine to allow their entry. The use of mechanical waste disposal units also helps. If conventional bins are used, they should be kept firmly covered and regularly emptied and cleaned.

Insecticidal sprays must not be allowed to come into contact with food and therefore must not be used in rooms where food is prepared. Electrically

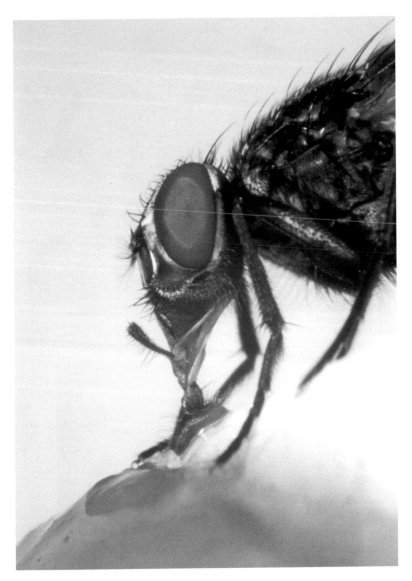

Close-up of a housefly on food

operated fly killers are suitable for food preparation areas. They consist of an ultraviolet light which attracts flies to a metal grid with an electric current running through it. The flies are electrocuted when they touch the metal grid and fall into a collecting tray underneath.

When deciding where to position electrocutors, it is important to ensure that dead flies from the collection tray cannot drop or be blown into food. A newer control system utilises ultraviolet light to attract flies to a hidden sticky film.

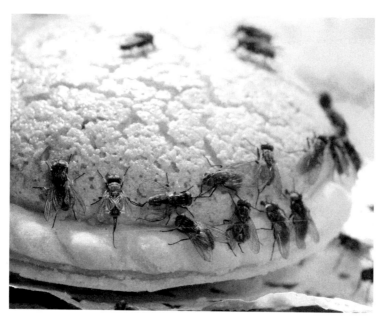

Houseflies

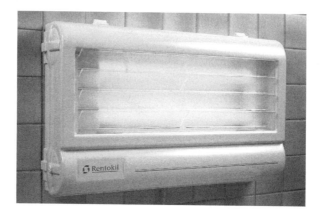

Electrically operated fly killer

Cockroaches

There are many different types of cockroach of varying sizes but only two are commonly found in the UK: the German cockroach and the oriental cockroach. The German cockroach is the smaller and is found in the kitchens of restaurants, hotels and industrial canteens. Typical hiding places are behind ovens and hot water pipes and around refrigerator motors. The larger oriental cockroach is usually found in the cooler and less humid parts of buildings such as basements, cellars and store rooms.

Cockroaches spread the bacteria that cause food poisoning and also those that cause dysentery and typhoid.

Their presence is not always detected at an early stage because they hide in crevices and cavities in the daytime and emerge to feed only at night. As they move around the kitchen in search of food they contaminate work surfaces, utensils, equipment and any uncovered food with pathogenic bacteria from their droppings and bodies.

An infestation by cockroaches can be recognised by their droppings and a characteristic and very unpleasant smell. It can be treated with insecticides but expert advice must be sought about the use of insecticides in food premises. Several treatments will be necessary because the eggs of the cockroach are protected by a capsule and do not hatch out for several months.

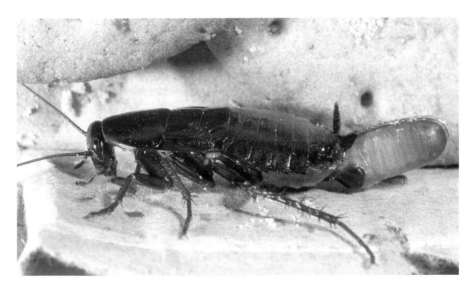

Oriental cockroach and egg capsule (actual size 22 mm)

Pharaoh's ants

Pharaoh's ants are small red-brown tropical ants. Infestations are found in warm, usually permanently heated premises, such as hospitals and bakeries. These ants carry many pathogenic bacteria including some capable of causing food poisoning. In hospitals, they are attracted to soiled dressings, toilets and drains and can therefore transmit many diseases. As with all pest infestations, professional advice must be sought as soon as an infestation is suspected.

Birds

The most common pest birds are sparrows, pigeons and starlings. They have been called 'flying mice' because their droppings, feathers and feet are heavily contaminated with food-poisoning bacteria. Birds can be removed from food premises by encouraging them to eat food mixed with a narcotic drug that causes deep sleep. They can then be removed from the premises and destroyed humanely. If any protected bird takes the bait, it can be revived and released unaffected.

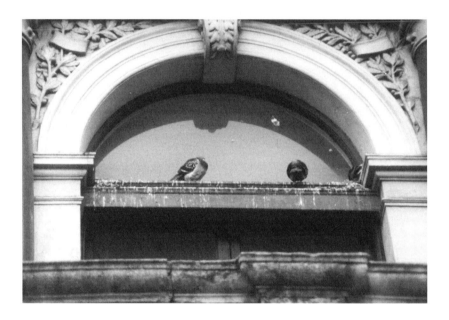

Stored product pests

Psocids (also called *booklice*) sometimes infest dry goods such as flour, milk powder, sugar or semolina. They are small (1–2 mm) grey or brown insects and are seen as dark specks in the food or in the folds of packaging. They are most likely to occur in dark areas of high humidity and rapidly increase in numbers in warm conditions.

To prevent a psocid infection:

❏ keep the kitchen and food storage cupboards well ventilated and dry

❏ check food cupboards regularly, using contents in 'best before' date order

❑   store vulnerable food like flour in washable covered containers

❑   check packaging and food on delivery to ensure it is not already infested.

If psocids have infested food, the best method of eliminating them is to remove and dispose of all infected food in an external dustbin. Thoroughly clean the cupboard using a dry cloth, by vacuuming, or by washing. Ensure the cupboard is completely dry before replacing any foods. This can be achieved by using a warm air blower like a hair dryer.

Other stored product pests include beetles, grain weevils and moths. Clean, well-ventilated and well-maintained stores combined with good stock rotation should stop any infestation. Several insecticides are suitable for use in food rooms if needed but specialist advice should be sought.

Summary

❑   Rats, mice, flies, cockroaches and Pharaoh's ants are the most common kitchen pests.

❑   Pests carry bacteria in their intestines, on their bodies and feet and can contaminate food or work surfaces with their droppings or by walking over them.

❑   If a pest infestation is suspected, expert advice must be sought.

20 FOOD SPOILAGE AND FOOD PRESERVATION

Food spoilage

All foods deteriorate on keeping. Changes in taste, texture, appearance and smell occur, frequently making the food inedible. The aim of food preservation is to reduce the rate at which this deterioration takes place. Most food spoilage is caused either by enzymes present in the food itself or by the growth of micro-organisms (bacteria, moulds or yeasts).

Enzymes

Immediately after slaughter or harvest, enzymes present in food start to break down the cell structure of the food. This process is known as *autolysis*. Autolysis causes a deterioration in the appearance and texture of the food and also makes the food more susceptible to attack by micro-organisms.

Microbial spoilage

Bacteria, moulds and yeasts are all capable of causing food spoilage when they grow and multiply in or on food. Spoilage bacteria are naturally present in foods such as milk and meat, yeasts are often present on fruit and mould spores are present in the air and start to germinate when they land on food. The type of spoilage will depend on a number of factors related to the food.

The pH of the food

The pH scale expresses the acidity or alkalinity of a substance. Water is neutral and has a pH of 7. Acid substances have a pH of less than 7 and alkaline substances have a pH greater than 7. Most foods are slightly acid. Egg white and some foods made with flour are weak alkalis.

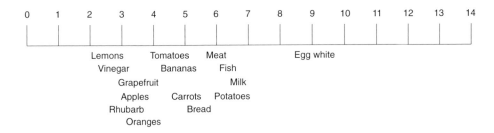

The pH scale

Bacteria are more likely to spoil foods with a near-neutral pH, for example milk, meat and fish.

Moulds and yeasts are more likely to spoil foods with a low pH, for example tomatoes, fruits, fruit juices.

The water activity of the food *(Aw)*

The water activity of a food is the amount of water that is available for microbial growth. The Aw of pure water is 1. Foods with plenty of available water have a high Aw (just less than 1). Foods with a high concentration of salt or sugar have a lower Aw (between 0.7 and 0.85) because the salt or sugar absorbs moisture and makes it unavailable for microbial growth.

Bacteria are more likely to spoil foods with a high Aw, for example milk, meat, eggs, fish.

Moulds are more likely to spoil foods with a lower Aw, for example bread, cheese, jam, cakes.

The composition of the food

Bacteria are more likely to spoil foods that are high in protein. Protein breakdown caused by bacteria results in the familiar unpleasant smells and tastes associated with 'off' meat or 'bad' eggs. Bacteria, moulds and yeasts use carbohydrates present in the food as a source of energy. As they multiply they produce acids, alcohols and gases that make the food taste sour, alcoholic or bubbly.

Food preservation

In order to preserve food it is necessary to either destroy the micro-organisms that are present on or in the food or to inhibit their growth in some way.

The preservation methods used fall into the following groups.

1   Low-temperature storage, for example refrigeration, freezing.

2   Use of high temperatures, for example cooking, pasteurisation and sterilisation (including canning).

3   Dehydration, for example drying, smoking, use of salt and sugar.

4   Use of chemical preservatives.

5   Vacuum packing.

6   Controlled atmosphere packaging.

7   Irradiation.

Use of low temperatures

Low-temperature preservation of food can be either short term (refrigeration) or long term (freezing).

Refrigeration

The correct running temperature of a refrigerator is 1–4°C. At this temperature most pathogens will not grow, except for Listeria (see p. 58) which is an exception and will grow slowly. Many spoilage bacteria and moulds will multiply slowly at refrigeration temperatures and consequently the flavour, taste and texture of food stored in a refrigerator will deteriorate but not as quickly as it would do at room temperature. It is therefore very important to observe the use-by dates on foods.

Freezing

The correct running temperature of a domestic freezer is –18°C. Micro-organisms will not multiply at this temperature but many will remain dormant. Moulds and yeasts are more likely to spoil frozen food than bacteria if the storage temperature is not low enough because they grow at a lower temperature and need less available water.

Enzymatic changes do take place very slowly, giving some deterioration in the quality of the food when it is stored for a long period of time. Vegetables should be blanched before freezing to destroy enzymes and reduce the number of bacteria present.

Rapid freezing of food will give a better quality product because it prevents the formation of large ice crystals. Most domestic freezers freeze food rather slowly and the large ice crystals formed cause a loss in texture of the food.

There are several different methods of commercial freezing but all of them aim to freeze the food as rapidly as possible. The shape and volume of the food usually dictate the method to be used.

Air blast freezing
The food is passed through a tunnel either on trolleys or on a continuous belt. Air at a temperature between −30 and −40°C circulates around the food, freezing it rapidly. This is the most commonly used method of commercial freezing and is suitable for large irregular-shaped foods such as chickens and also for boxed meals.

Plate freezing
The food is placed between metal plates through which a refrigerant circulates. This method is suitable for fairly flat, regular-shaped foods such as burgers. They are often packed in their cartons before being frozen.

Fluidised bed freezing
The food is placed on a perforated belt which is passed through a tunnel. Freezing air is forced up through the perforations, allowing each item to be individually frozen. This method is used for peas and other small items.

Immersion (cryogenic) freezing
The food is dipped into a refrigerant such as liquid nitrogen which freezes it very rapidly. This is an expensive method and is used for luxury items such as raspberries and prawns.

Use of high temperatures

The main reason for cooking food is to make it more palatable, but cooking also destroys many of the pathogenic bacteria and many of those that cause spoilage. Pasteurisation and sterilisation are the most common methods of preserving food by the application of heat. Pasteurisation is a short-term method of preservation and results in less change in the quality and nutritive value of the food than sterilisation, which is a long-term method and affects the quality and nutritive value of the food to a greater extent.

Pasteurisation
This mild heat process is designed to reduce the number of spoilage micro-organisms and destroy the pathogenic ones.

Milk was originally pasteurised to destroy the bacteria that cause tuberculosis. It is heated to 72°C for 15 seconds and then cooled rapidly to below 10°C. This process destroys Salmonella and Campylobacter, which may be present in raw milk, and also destroys some of the spoilage bacteria, so the milk will keep for longer.

By law, liquid egg and ice cream mix must be pasteurised in order to destroy Salmonella and any other pathogens present. A number of different combinations of time and temperature are used to achieve pasteurisation of ice cream – 65.6°C for 30 minutes, 71.1°C for 10 minutes, 79.4°C for 15 seconds, followed by rapid cooling. A high temperature for a shorter time generally results in a better product with less loss of flavour. More heat is needed to pasteurise ice cream than milk because ice cream is rich in sugar and fat which give bacteria some protection.

Liquid egg is pasteurised at 64.4°C for $2\frac{1}{2}$ minutes and then cooled rapidly. The temperature at which it is pasteurised must be below 65°C in order to prevent protein coagulation.

Sterilisation

This heat process is designed to kill all micro-organisms and their spores. Milk is sterilised by heating it in sealed bottles under pressure to 112°C for 15 minutes.

Milk that has been sterilised has a 'cooked' flavour but it will keep for several years at room temperature.

Ultra-high temperature (UHT) treatment

This heat process will destroy all micro-organisms but not all spores. The milk is heated to 132°C for 1 second and then cooled rapidly and aseptically packed (a method of packing which does not allow the entry of any micro-organisms). UHT milk will keep for six months or more at room temperature and it has a better flavour than sterilised milk.

Canning

Canning is a widely used method of food preservation. The food is put in a metal can, sealed so that no further micro-organisms can enter the food and then sterilised. The most important consideration is to ensure that any spores of *Clostridium botulinum* are destroyed, since this pathogen would thrive in canned foods because of the absence of oxygen (see p. 57).

The combination of time and temperature required to sterilise the food in the can depend on:

❏   the size of the can

❏   the consistency of the food

❏   the pH of the food.

Sufficient heat must be applied to sterilise the food in the centre of the can, allowing for the fact that heat has to penetrate from the outside to the

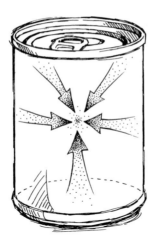

The heat has to penetrate to the food in the centre of the can

centre. A large can of solid food, for example corned beef, will take longer to sterilise than a small can of liquid food, such as soup. *Clostridium botulinum* and many other pathogens do not grow in very acid foods (pH less than 4.5) and hence acid foods require less heat treatment than near-neutral foods in order to achieve sterilisation.

Aseptic canning
Aseptic canning is a variation on the standard canning process whereby the cans and the bulk product are sterilised separately and then filled in conditions that prevent the entry of any further micro-organisms. Aseptic canning is used for foods that are sensitive to heat, such as dairy custards and other milk products, which would be burnt at the surface in the standard canning process. It is a particularly useful method for large cans.

Pasteurised canned hams
Some catering-sized cans of ham are pasteurised rather than sterilised because the high temperatures required for sterilisation would cause shrinkage and loss of flavour. The saltiness of the product also helps to preserve it but since some micro-organisms are present, pasteurised canned hams must be stored in a refrigerator. The manufacturer's storage instructions appear on the label and must be followed.

Spoilage of canned foods

Once a can has been opened the food in it must be treated as fresh food and stored in a refrigerator. Uneaten food must not be left in the can because it absorbs tin from the can, particularly if it is an acid food, such as tomatoes.

Unopened cans sometimes develop bulges at the ends due to gas produced inside. These are known as 'blown' cans and must not be used. The gas has probably been produced by bacteria, which means that either the can was understerilised or that it is a faulty can that has allowed bacteria to enter after sterilisation. Any other cans from the same batch (as indicated by the code on the end of the can) must not be used without discussing the problem with the manufacturer or an environmental health officer. Similarly, rusty or badly dented cans should not be used as it is possible that there will be a small opening somewhere in the can.

Dehydration

Dehydration reduces the moisture content (*Aw*) of foods to levels at which micro-organisms cannot grow (about 0.6). Dehydrated foods are not sterile and bacteria can survive in them for many years. When dehydrated foods are reconstituted, any bacteria present will start to multiply. If the reconstituted food is not going to be used immediately, it should be refrigerated.

Drying of food causes some irreversible changes to the food and the reconstituted product generally has a poorer flavour and texture and suffers greater loss of nutritive value than if the food had been frozen. The advantage of drying food is that it does not need any special storage conditions other than being in air-tight packs and kept dry. In hot climates sun-drying is still practised, particularly for figs, currants and tomatoes. There are several methods used for commercial drying of food.

Tunnel drying and fluidised bed drying

These techniques involve passing the food through a tunnel while hot air is blown across or from underneath the food. They are used for fruits and vegetables, which must be blanched before dehydration to stop enzyme activity during storage.

Spray drying and roller drying

These techniques are suitable for liquid foods. In spray drying the liquid is sprayed into a stream of hot air. The moisture in the droplets evaporates rapidly, resulting in the retention of good flavour, colour and nutritive value. Roller drying involves covering a revolving heated drum with a paste of the food to be dried. When the moisture content has been reduced to the desired level a scraper removes the food from the drum. Spray drying usually gives a better quality product than roller drying.

Accelerated freeze drying

In this technique the food is frozen first and then heated under vacuum. The ice is converted to water vapour (*sublimation*). Accelerated freeze drying affects the structure of the food less than other drying methods and gives a better quality product when reconstituted.

Smoking

Smoking is an ancient method of food preservation but is now used mainly to give the food a characteristic flavour and texture rather than as a method of preservation. The drying effect on the surface of the food and several of the compounds in the smoke will inhibit the growth of some micro-organisms. Smoked foods must always be refrigerated.

Salt and sugar

High concentrations of salt and sugar in food make the water in the food unavailable for microbial growth. Certain foods can therefore be preserved by the addition of salt or sugar. The preservative effect may be only partial and is often used with other preservative methods such as refrigeration.

Salt is used in the curing of foods such as pork and fish. The curing medium is a brine, containing sodium chloride (salt), sodium nitrate and sodium nitrite. The food is immersed in the brine or the brine is injected into the food. Salted meat and fish have a characteristic flavour and colour.

Sugar is used mainly to preserve fruit in various forms such as jams, marmalades and crystallised fruits.

Chemical preservatives

Several chemicals are widely used in the preservation of food.

Acetic acid (vinegar) is used to preserve vegetables such as onions, cabbages, cauliflowers and gherkins, as well as for the manufacture of products such as chutney and salad cream. Adding vinegar lowers the pH of the food so that it is too acid for bacterial growth.

Making *yoghurt* is a traditional method of preserving milk. Bacteria that convert lactose to lactic acid are added to the milk to lower its pH.

Sulphur dioxide is added to many foods to help preserve them, including sausages, dried fruit, beer and wine. Sulphur dioxide in food is converted to sulphurous acid, which lowers the pH and hence has a preservative effect.

Sodium nitrate and sodium nitrite are used in the curing process and are also added to canned and vacuum-packed meats. Sodium nitrite very effectively inhibits the growth of *Clostridium botulinum*, but in recent years there has been some controversy over its use. It is thought that the ingestion of nitrites might possibly lead to the development of some types of cancer. It is, however, unlikely that the quantities used in food present any significant risk.

Vacuum packing

Vacuum packing foods stops the growth of aerobic micro-organisms such as moulds and some spoilage bacteria but will not stop the growth of anaerobic bacteria. Vacuum packing hard cheeses prevents mould spoilage on the surface and the low moisture content of hard cheese inhibits bacterial growth. Vacuum packing will not inhibit the growth of *Clostridium botulinum* and therefore where pathogenic bacteria including *Clostridium botulinum* may be present, for example in meats, it must be used in conjunction with other methods of preservation, such as refrigeration or the addition of nitrites.

Controlled atmosphere packaging

Carbon dioxide is sometimes used in conjunction with refrigeration to reduce the rate of spoilage of fresh meat, fruits, vegetables and eggs. The optimum concentration of carbon dioxide in the atmosphere varies depending on the type of food. Too much carbon dioxide in the atmosphere can cause tissue damage and produce 'off' flavours.

Irradiation

Irradiating food with gamma rays is an effective method of destroying both pathogenic and spoilage micro-organisms in foods such as raw chicken, fruit, vegetables, spices, shellfish and cereals. Spores and toxins are unaffected at the levels used. There is very little change, if any, in the taste or texture of the food as a result of irradiation. Irradiated food is considered to be perfectly safe to eat but there is a great reluctance by members of the public to accept foods that have been treated in this way. Any food that has been irradiated must be labelled accordingly.

Irradiation can be used to destroy Salmonella in animal feeds. If all feeds were treated in this way there would be a significant reduction in the number of animals carrying Salmonella. The expense of the process is the main prohibitive factor.

Summary

❏ Enzymes, bacteria, moulds and yeasts all contribute to food spoilage.

❏ The type of spoilage depends on the pH, the Aw and the composition of the food.

❏ Preservation methods involve the use of one or more of the following: low temperatures; high temperatures; dehydration; chemicals; controlled atmospheres or physical methods.

21 FOOD HAZARD ANALYSIS

Over the last 20 years the Hazard Analysis and Critical Control Points system (HACCP–pronounced *hassup*) has been developed and is now widely used in the food industry to help businesses ensure that they are producing and selling food which is safe to eat. This 'prevention is better than cure' approach to food hygiene is a shift from the traditional practice of making investigations after a complaint or problem has occurred and trying to ensure it does not happen again to the practice of identifying potential problems before they arise and eliminating the factors which may cause the problems.

Two examples of potential hazards and the way to control them before they become problems are as follows:

1   *Hazard*–metal object in food.
    Control – using a metal detector on a factory line to detect and remove metal.

2   *Hazard*–large numbers of bacteria present in food after refrigeration.
    Control – reading and recording refrigeration temperatures at regular intervals and taking appropriate action if the readings are too high.

Before applying a HACCP system to a food manufacturing business it must already be operating with high standards of hygiene and the following good practices must be in place:

❑   Adequate cleaning and disinfection of equipment.

❑   High standards of personal hygiene of food handlers.

❑   A satisfactory system of pest control.

❑   Appropriate food hygiene training given to all employees.

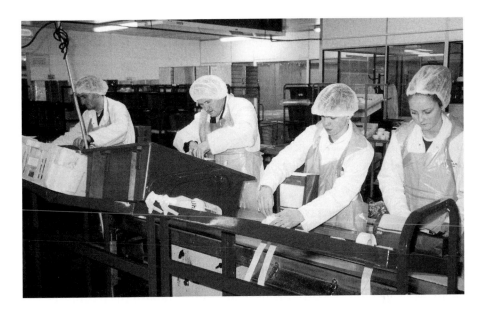

Setting up an HACCP system

The HACCP team may be small and consist of one or two people or it may be large, depending on the scale of operation under review. It may be enough to have one or two people who know the business well and have the necessary expertise and knowledge of food hygiene or it may be necessary to include people with additional skills such as engineering or microbiology.

The HACCP team considers each step in the manufacturing process from the purchase of raw materials through each of the stages in factory production to the sale and even the storage after purchase of the food. The team draws up a flow chart which identifies each stage of the production and supply process.

The main stages in drawing up an HACCP scheme are:

1 conduct a hazard analysis

2 determine the critical control points

3 monitor the critical control points and take corrective action if necessary

4 review the scheme.

Hazard analysis

What is a hazard? A food hazard is anything that could potentially make food harmful to eat. It can be physical, chemical or microbiological. The most likely hazards in a food production process are:

❏ presence of food-poisoning bacteria, foreign bodies or unacceptable levels of pesticides in ingredients when arriving at the factory

❏ contamination of the food with bacteria during the manufacturing process

❏ keeping the food in suitable conditions for rapid bacterial growth

❏ contamination of the food with foreign bodies such as glass, chemicals or metal during the production process

❏ contamination by pests.

Every food business will have different hazards depending on the type of food being prepared and the method of preparation.

Determining the critical control points

Having identified the hazards, the next step is to establish the risk or the likelihood of the hazard happening. If the risk is significant, control measures must be introduced at points where they will be effective. These points are known as *critical control points*.

The checks necessary at critical control points are most likely to concern:

❏ detection and removal of foreign bodies

❏ time and temperature of storage

❏ personal hygiene

❏ cross-contamination

❏ cleaning and disinfection.

For each critical control point (CCP) there must be a target level for the control in place and a tolerance which is the extent to which the target level can vary with little or no risk of causing a problem. If the measurement falls outside the tolerance of the target level, remedial action must be taken straight away. A set of procedures is laid down which must be followed in order to decide what must happen to the food. It may be necessary to destroy that batch of food.

CCP	Target	Tolerance
Hot holding of food	30 minutes	+/–5 minutes
Metal in food	All metal detected	None
Storage of high-risk food	3°C	+/–2°C

When trying to decide where exactly in the food preparation process the critical control point occurs, it is helpful to consider whether action at a later stage in the process will remove the hazard or not. If action at a later stage will not remove the hazard, then that point in the process is a critical control point.

Monitoring and corrective action

Once the critical control points have been identified, it is possible to put in checks at the appropriate stages in production that will stop the hazard occurring. For each critical control point it should be determined:

- ❑ *what* checks should be made
- ❑ *when* they should be made
- ❑ *who* is to do them.

Many of the checks made are time and temperature measurements and visual assessments. All checks must be recorded and signed by the person who has made them. It is very important to establish when further action is necessary and who is to take it otherwise efficient recording of information is pointless.

Review

HACCP is an excellent system which helps to produce safe food. It must be regularly reviewed and modified if it is to remain effective. When new procedures or equipment are introduced, the hazard analysis must be revised. Similarly, the production of a different type of food will mean that the hazard analysis must be reviewed. Even when there have been no changes, reviews must take place at least annually.

Hazard analysis and the catering industry

The 1995 Food Safety (General Food Hygiene) Regulations state that the proprietor of a food business must carry out a food hazard analysis but they do not demand a fully documented HACCP system. Full HACCP systems are widely used in food factories but their use is not appropriate in a kitchen serving a restaurant because the types and methods of preparing food are so variable. However, the principles of HACCP can be applied to the catering industry to very good effect. By grouping similar dishes together it is possible to work out potential hazards and take steps to monitor and control them.

For example, in the preparation and cooking of chicken (or any other high-risk food) for serving at a cold buffet the hazards most likely to occur are the growth of pathogenic micro-organisms due to poor temperature control and cross-contamination. The following table suggests the questions which should be asked and the checks to be made at each stage of the food preparation process.

Step	Monitoring
Purchase and delivery	Checks on the supplier
	Specification for product quality
	Satisfactory wrapping
	Temperature and condition on delivery
Storage	Time between delivery and storage
	Can cross-contamination occur?
	Stock rotation/date codes
	Pest control
Cooking	Complete thawing if originally frozen
	Adequate cooking-centre temperature, at least 75°C
Preparation	Cleaning and disinfection of preparation surfaces
	Length of time at room temperature
	Cross-contamination?
	Personal hygiene of food handlers
Cooling	Length of time at room temperature
Service	Length of time on display at room temperature

It is very important to have an 'action plan' if any of the readings taken or checks made are unsatisfactory. If the temperature of the chicken in the refrigerator is consistently higher than 5°C this information should not only be recorded but employees should know what action to take to correct the problem or whom they should inform. There may be several reasons for the high temperature of the food and the following questions should be asked.

❑ Is the refrigerator too full?

❑ Is the temperature of the food too high when it is put in the refrigerator?

❑ Does the refrigerator need repairing or replacing?

A written record should be made of potential hazards, checks and controls because it is difficult to apply controls consistently if there is no documentation. It is also useful to have written evidence of them to show an environmental health officer during an inspection and would be very useful if a defence of due diligence were ever necessary (see p. 144).

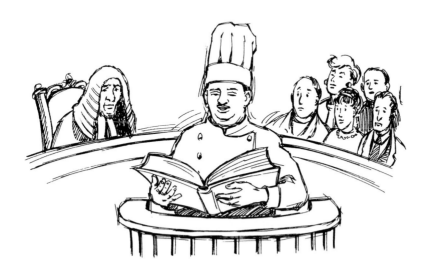

Summary

❑ HACCP systems are widely used in food factories.

❑ By following the principles of HACCP, a restaurant can improve the quality of foods served and have a greatly reduced chance of causing food poisoning.

22 FOOD HYGIENE LEGISLATION

Laws on food safety exist to ensure that people are provided with food which is safe to eat. Food safety legislation is a complex subject and a local environmental health officer should be consulted if help is needed with the interpretation of any aspect of the legislation.

Legislation takes several different forms:

❏ *Acts of Parliament.* These are generally concerned with the principles of the law.

❏ *Regulations and Orders.* These are more specific and may relate to a particular type of food business, e.g. butcher's shops, or to a specific commodity, e.g. shellfish, dairy products.

❏ *Local Acts or Bylaws.* These are adopted and enforced by the local authority and concern its area only, e.g. places where street trading is permitted.

Main legislation

Food businesses in England and Wales are covered by the following legislation:

❏ The Food Safety Act 1990 (see p. 141)

❏ The Food Safety (General Food Hygiene) Regulations 1995 (see p. 144)

❏ The Food Safety (Temperature Control) Regulations 1995 parts I, II and IV (see p. 146)

❏ The Food Premises (Registration) Regulations 1991–1997 (see p. 147)

❏ The Food Safety (General Food Hygiene) (Butchers' Shops) Amendment Regulations 2000 (see p. 148).

Food businesses in Scotland are covered by the following legislation:

❑ The Food Safety Act 1990 (see below)

❑ The Food Safety (General Food Hygiene) Regulations 1995 (see p. 144)

❑ The Food Safety (Temperature Control) Regulations 1995, Parts I, III and IV (see p. 146)

❑ The Food Safety (Registration) Regulations 1991–1997 (see p. 147)

❑ The Food Safety (General Food Hygiene) (Butchers' Shops) Amendment (Scotland) Regulations 2000 (see p. 147).

Food businesses in Northern Ireland are covered by the following legislation.

❑ The Food Safety (Northern Ireland) Order 1991

❑ The Food Premises (General Food Hygiene) Regulations (Northern Ireland) 1995

❑ The Food Safety (Temperature Control) Regulations (Northern Ireland) 1995

❑ The Food Premises (Registration) Regulations (Northern Ireland) 1992 and Amendments 1997.

Food Safety Act 1990

This Act is concerned with the safety of food from farm production to the point when it is sold. It is an offence to sell or possess for sale food that:

❑ is not of the nature, substance or quality demanded

❑ is unfit to eat either because it is contaminated with pathogenic micro-organisms or because it contains poisonous chemicals or foreign bodies

❑ has false or misleading labelling or advertisement

❑ does not meet food safety requirements

❑ is rendered injurious to health

❑ is unfit for human consumption.

Anyone who owns, manages or works in a food business must adhere to this legislation. This includes people who transport, pack and store food and not just those who prepare it. All types of food businesses are included: anything from an expensive restaurant or large supermarket to a stall in a village hall or a vending machine.

Food safety legislation is enforced by local authorities through the work of environmental health officers and trading standards officers. Environmental health officers deal with hygiene of food premises and cases where food is contaminated with micro-organisms or for any other reason is unfit for human consumption. Trading standards officers deal with the labelling of food, its composition and most cases of chemical contamination.

In Scotland, environmental health officers and other authorised officers deal with all food hygiene and food standards matters. Trading standards officers have no role in these matters in Scotland.

Under the provisions of the Food Safety Act, an authorised officer (usually an environmental health officer) may enter food premises at any reasonable time to inspect them.

Inspection of premises

Environmental health officers or other authorised officers inspect all food businesses on a regular basis and will make extra visits if there is any reason to suspect that premises or practices are unhygienic. The officer identifies the risks attached to each particular business and considers the effectiveness of the systems employed to control potential problems. It is useful to have a brief written explanation of the systems in place to show the environmental health officer (see Hazard analysis, p. 137).

The main points that the environmental health officer considers are as follows.

1 The food safety management system.

2 Risks of contamination.

3 Staff training.

4 Personal hygiene.

5 Are the premises clean and well maintained?

6 Are the premises suitable for the scale of operation?

7 Is there adequate refrigeration space?

8 Is the food storage space adequate?

9 Is there an adequate number of sinks and wash hand-basins?

10 Are the premises well lit and ventilated?

11 Are all the work surfaces clean and of suitable material?

12 Are all the utensils and equipment clean?

13 Are the methods of refuse disposal suitable?

14 Are there any signs of pest infestation?

15 Are the toilet facilities clean?

16 Is there a suitable cleaning schedule in operation?

17 Do the staff:
- ❑ keep and prepare raw and cooked food separately?
- ❑ handle food as little as possible?
- ❑ ensure food is kept cold (below 8°C) or hot (above 63°C)?
- ❑ wear clean washable overalls?

18 Are the staff aware that:
- ❑ they should not smoke whilst they are in a food room?
- ❑ they should report any illness, especially vomiting or diarrhoea?
- ❑ they should cover any cuts with a detectable waterproof plaster?

After an inspection the environmental health officer might write informally to the proprietor of the business asking him or her to put right any problems which have come to light during the inspection. If the offences are more serious the officer may take one of the following actions:

1 Issue an *Improvement Notice*, which requests that certain measures are taken in order to comply with food hygiene legislation. A specified time limit is set for the improvements to be made which will be at least a fortnight.

2 Prosecute the proprietor for a breach of the food hygiene regulations. In Scotland, a report would be sent to the Procurator Fiscal who would decide whether to prosecute. If the court feels that public health is at risk it will impose a *Prohibition Order*, which closes all of the business or the part of the business that does not comply with the regulations.

3 Issue an *Emergency Prohibition Notice*. If the offence poses an immediate risk to health, the environmental health officer can close the premises immediately for three days by issuing an Emergency Prohibition Notice. The matter is taken before a court within three days. If the court agrees that the offence poses an immediate risk to health it will issue an *Emergency Prohibition Order*, which keeps the premises closed until the necessary improvements have been made.

To lift a Prohibition Order or an Emergency Prohibition Order and reopen the premises the proprietor must apply to the environmental health department for a *Certificate of Compliance*, stating that the risk to health has been removed.

Food hygiene offences are usually brought to a magistrates' court or in Scotland, a sheriff court without a jury, where the penalty for contravening the legislation is a maximum fine of £20 000 (Food Safety Act 1990). Food hygiene offences in England and Wales can be brought to a Crown court. There is no maximum fine in a Crown court and a prison sentence of up to two years may be imposed. In Scotland, a sheriff court with a jury has the same powers.

Due diligence defence

If a person who is responsible for food safety commits an offence and is prosecuted, it may be possible to establish a defence of due diligence if that person can prove that:

❑ the offence was the fault of another person

❑ he or someone he trusted had carried out all the necessary checks

❑ he had no reason to believe that his omission or action would amount to an offence.

A due diligence defence might be appropriate if, for example, a caterer was supplied with ready-prepared meals which turned out to cause food poisoning. The caterer would have to prove that he had taken all reasonable precautions to avoid this situation by carrying out all necessary checks on the method of production and by obtaining details of storage and transportation temperatures of the food before delivery. Written records of the date and types of checks made would be very valuable in such a defence.

The Food Safety (General Food Hygiene) Regulations 1995

The main requirements of this legislation are as follows.

1 Hygiene standards

All businesses must operate hygienically. Rooms where food is prepared, treated or processed should:

❑ be cleaned and maintained in good repair

❑ have surface finishes which are easy to clean and, where necessary, disinfect

❑ have an adequate supply of drinking water

❑ have adequate facilities, including hot and cold water, for washing food and equipment

❑ have adequate hand-washing facilities

❑ have suitable controls in place to protect against pests

❑ have adequate natural and/or artificial light

❑ have sufficient natural and/or artificial ventilation. Filters must be accessible for cleaning

❑ provide clean lavatories which do not lead directly into food rooms.

These basic minimum hygiene standards apply to all food businesses but for example, whether a surface is cleaned or disinfected and how often will depend on whether it is being used for the preparation of high-risk or low-risk foods.

All food handlers must maintain a high standard of personal hygiene. They should:

- ❏   wash hands frequently when handling food
- ❏   wear clean overalls
- ❏   never smoke whilst preparing food
- ❏   report to the manager any illnesses, particularly vomiting, diarrhoea and infected wounds.

It is expected that all food handlers will observe these rules, but for example, the frequency of hand washing will vary depending on whether high-risk or low-risk foods are being handled.

2 Hazard analysis

Managers of food businesses must identify the food safety hazards and critical control points in their particular business and devise procedures to control these risks (see Chapter 21).

The Food Safety (General Food Hygiene) Regulations 1995 do not demand a fully documented hazard analysis system but the proprietor has a legal obligation to establish a system and keep it under review. An outline of the checks in place for each process in the business would be useful to show an officer during an inspection and may be very important in establishing a defence of due diligence if necessary.

To help food businesses comply with the Food Safety (General Food Hygiene) Regulations 1995 and the Food Safety (Temperature Control) Regulations 1995, the government and representatives of the food industry have produced a series of industry guides to good hygiene practice. These are official guides to the Regulations which have been written in response to Article 5 of the EC Directive on the Hygiene of Foodstuffs. The guides are not legally binding but Food Authorities must give the guides due consideration when enforcing the Regulations. The guides cover the following sectors of the food industry:

1   Catering

2   Retail

3   Baking

4   Wholesale

5   Markets and fairs.

3 Training

The Food Safety (General Food Hygiene) Regulations 1995 put the responsibility for hygiene training of food handlers onto the owner of a food business. The extent of training will be different for each individual depending on the type of food they handle. Staff who handle the high-risk foods will need more training than those who handle low-risk foods. Special arrangements may have to be made for those employees whose first language is not English.

Staff may be trained 'in house' or alternatively can attend a food hygiene training course.

Chapter X of the Food Safety (General Food Hygiene) Regulations 1995 requires that '…food handlers engaged in the food business are supervised and instructed and/or trained in food hygiene matters commensurate with their work activities'. The various industry guides to good hygiene practice contain much useful information to help food businesses comply with this requirement.

It is useful to keep a record of training given to each member of staff which is signed by the person concerned.

Food Safety (Temperature Control) Regulations 1995 (England and Wales)

All food likely to support the growth of pathogenic bacteria or the formation of toxins must be stored at a temperature below 8°C. If a food which normally supports the growth of micro-organisms is stored above 8°C, the owner of the food business must be able to offer a scientific assessment (a microbiological analysis by a qualified scientist) of the safety of the food under the conditions in which it is stored. If the food is to be served hot it must be kept at a temperature of 63°C or above. Food which is about to be served hot may be kept at a temperature below 63°C for a maximum period of two hours. Food which is about to be served cold may be kept at a temperature above 8°C for a maximum of four hours.

The Food Safety (Temperature Control) Regulations 1995 (Scotland)

Food which is likely to support the growth of pathogenic bacteria or the formation of toxins must be stored in a refrigerator or a cool ventilated place. The various industry guides to good hygiene practice advise on good practice as no temperature is specified in law. Alternatively the food must be kept above 63°C. There are exceptions to allow food to be prepared, exposed for sale, sold to a consumer or to be cooled.

Food which is being reheated must reach a temperature of not less than 82°C.

Finally, there is an over-riding requirement that all foods, whether raw or finished products, are not kept at a temperature which would result in a risk to health.

The Food Premises (Registration) Regulations 1991–1997

Food premises, including mobile premises, must be registered with their local authority if they operate five or more days in five consecutive weeks. New businesses must apply for registration at least 28 days before they open. There is no charge for registration although failing to register may result in a fine. The local authority cannot refuse registration.

The Food Safety (General Food Hygiene) (Butchers' Shops) Amendment Regulations 2000

These Regulations apply in England and Wales. Any shop, including mobile shops and market stalls, which handles and sells unwrapped raw meat together with ready-to-eat food needs a licence. This licence is issued by the local authority subject to satisfactory hygiene conditions being in place. It is also a requirement that the method of operation of the business is documented and is in line with the principles of the HACCP approach. A comprehensive staff training plan must also be in place. The charge for the licence is £100.

The Food Safety (General Food Hygiene) (Butchers' Shops) Amendment (Scotland) Regulations 2000

All butchers' shops in Scotland which deal with unwrapped raw meat and ready-to-eat, including wrapped, food require a licence. In order to obtain a licence the business must comply with these Regulations. The Food Safety (General Food Hygiene) Regulations 1995 and The Food Safety (Temperature Control) Regulations 1995 and have all staff trained to at least the standards of the Elementary Food Hygiene Course. Supervisors must be trained to at least the Intermediate Food Hygiene Course level.

In addition, the business must have HACCP procedures in place or comply with a list of additional conditions contained in the Regulations.

Investigation of an outbreak of food poisoning

Any person who suspects that they are suffering from food poisoning should go to their doctor who is obliged to inform the local authority if he thinks his patient is suffering from food poisoning.

Cases of food poisoning are investigated by an environmental health officer. All patients are questioned about their symptoms, what food they have eaten in the last 48 hours and where it was eaten. Samples of their faeces are sent to a public health laboratory for bacteriological examination. If staphylococcal food poisoning is suspected, samples of vomit may be sent for analysis.

If most of the patients bought their food at a particular shop or restaurant, the environmental health officer will visit the premises and carry out an inspection and collect samples of any remaining suspect food.

A faecal sample may be taken from anyone who is in contact with food at the premises and if staphylococcal infection is suspected, nose, throat and skin swabs may be taken. Working surfaces and equipment may also be swabbed. All the samples are taken to the public health laboratory where they are checked to see whether they carry any bacteria identical to those isolated from the patient.

If the cause of the outbreak is discovered, appropriate action will be taken to ensure that no further outbreaks occur. Food handlers who are suffering from the same illness will be excluded from work. They may return to work 48 hours after the vomiting and diarrhoea have ceased provided no medication is being taken to control the symptoms. If the food handler is infected with *Salmonella typhi* or *S. paratyphi*, exclusion from work continues until six consecutive negative stool samples taken at 14-day intervals are obtained. The local authority will pay the food handler's wages for the period he is excluded from work but he will be prosecuted if he returns to work during that period.

PRACTICAL FOOD HYGIENE

PERSONAL HYGIENE

- **Wash hands often -** especially:
  - before touching any food
  - after touching raw food, eg meat and poultry
  - after going to the toilet
- Wear clean protective clothing
- Don't smoke or spit in food handling areas
- Don't cough or sneeze over food
- Cover cuts and sores with waterproof dressings

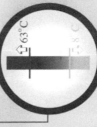

ILLNESS

- **Tell your supervisor if you feel unwell,** or if you have been ill while on holiday, as you could contaminate food. Always tell them if you have:
  - diarrhoea and/or vomiting, or
  - infected wounds, or any other skin infection
- **Don't handle food if you have:**
  - diarrhoea and/or vomiting
  - infected sores or cuts, unless they are well covered to prevent contamination

TRAINING, INSTRUCTION AND SUPERVISION

- **Food handlers must by law be supervised and instructed and/or trained in food hygiene matters,** so that any food handled is safe for the consumer

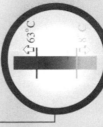

KEEPING FOOD SAFE FROM CONTAMINATION

- **Protect food and ingredients from contamination - at all times**
- Clean and routinely disinfect all work surfaces and equipment that come into contact with food
- Use potable (drinking) water to wash food
- Clean and disinfect utensils after contact with raw food - ideally use separate utensils when preparing raw and ready to eat food
- Keep raw food, especially meat, separate from ready to eat food

TEMPERATURE CONTROL

- **Good temperature control is essential**
- Keep all food requiring temperature control[†] (eg products containing meat, fish, eggs, milk, cooked vegetables and pulses):
  - **CHILLED - at or below 8°C, or**
  - **HOT - at or above 63°C**
- When cooking foods ensure they are cooked thoroughly
- Reheat foods until piping hot throughout
- Cool food for refrigeration quickly - ideally within 90 minutes of preparation

[†] Legal requirements are contained in The Food Safety (Temperature Control) Regulations 1995.

IF YOU WORK WITH FOOD THE LAW REQUIRES GOOD HYGIENE PRACTICES TO ENSURE FOOD IS SAFE TO EAT. THIS POSTER GIVES PRACTICAL ADVICE ON THE LAW AND YOUR RESPONSIBILITIES.

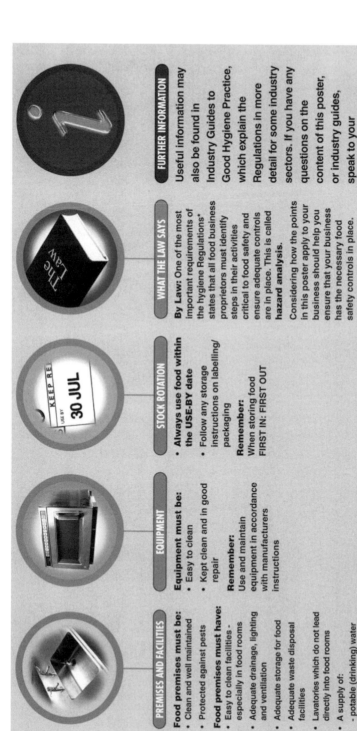

PREMISES AND FACILITIES

Food premises must be:
- Clean and well maintained
- Protected against pests

Food premises must have:
- Easy to clean facilities - especially in food rooms
- Adequate drainage, lighting and ventilation
- Adequate storage for food
- Adequate waste disposal facilities
- Lavatories which do not lead directly into food rooms
- A supply of:
  - potable (drinking) water
  - hot water
- Sinks for washing food and equipment

And separate:
- Facilities for washing hands

EQUIPMENT

Equipment must be:
- Easy to clean
- Kept clean and in good repair

Remember:
Use and maintain equipment in accordance with manufacturers instructions

STOCK ROTATION

- Always use food within the **USE-BY** date
- Follow any storage instructions on labelling/packaging

Remember:
When storing food
FIRST IN: FIRST OUT

WHAT THE LAW SAYS

By Law: One of the most important requirements of the hygiene Regulations* states that all food business proprietors must identify steps in their activities critical to food safety and ensure adequate controls are in place. This is called **hazard analysis.**

Considering how the points in this poster apply to your business should help you ensure that your business has the necessary food safety controls in place.

FURTHER INFORMATION

Useful information may also be found in Industry Guides to Good Hygiene Practice, which explain the Regulations in more detail for some industry sectors. If you have any questions on the content of this poster, or industry guides, speak to your supervisor or local environmental health department.

*This poster summarises the main requirements of The Food Safety (General Food Hygiene) Regulations 1995. The information contained is only advisory - individual food premises are responsible for checking how the Regulations apply in practice to them.

© Crown Copyright
Produced by Department of Health
10115 HEF 17Ak Mar 97 SA (02)
CHLORINE FREE PAPER

23 FOOD HYGIENE, TRAVEL AND TOURISM

Tourism is a growing industry. Overseas travel is becoming increasingly popular, not only in the number of people travelling abroad but also in the variety of destinations visited. In the year 2000 there were approximately 660 million international travellers.

Unfortunately many people experience illness when they travel abroad. A recent survey showed that 10% of tourists visiting southern Europe suffered from diarrhoea during their stay and 50% of tourists to Latin America, North Africa, India and Nepal suffered illness. In most cases of holiday diarrhoea, people come to no serious harm and recover completely apart from a ruined holiday or an interrupted business trip. But for a few the illness will give rise to prolonged ill health or may even be fatal.

Travellers are particularly susceptible to food poisoning and food-borne diseases because they are exposed to food and drinking water which contains pathogens not previously met in their home country. This puts them at greater risk than the local population. The risk is greater for travellers staying in accommodation with primitive washing and toilet facilities and eating in local restaurants than for those staying in five-star hotels but even food handlers in 5-star hotels are not always reliable!

Another factor is that elderly people travel regularly and they are more susceptible to food poisoning than healthy young adults.

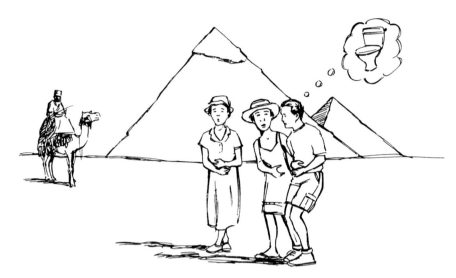

The following illnesses can be contracted as a result of eating contaminated food or drinking contaminated water. Some are caused by bacteria, others by viruses, toxins, protozoa or parasitic worms.

Illness	Caused by
Traveller's diarrhoea	Bacteria (*E. coli*)
Typhoid fever	Bacteria (*Salmonella typhi*)
Paratyphoid fever	Bacteria (*Salmonella paratyphi*)
Dysentery	Bacteria (Shigella)
Vibrio parahaemolyticus food poisoning	Bacteria (*V. parahaemolyticus*)
Brucellosis	Bacteria (*Brucella abortus*)
Scombrotoxic fish poisoning	Toxins
Paralytic shellfish poisoning	Toxins
Ciguatera poisoning	Toxins
Giardiasis	Protozoa
Cryptosporidiosis	Protozoa
Amoebic dysentery	Protozoa
Hepatits A and hepatitis E	Virus
Polio	Virus
Intestinal roundworm infection	Nematodes, e.g. *Ascaris lumbricoides* – Giant human roundworm *Trichuris trichiura* – Human whipworm
Trichinosis	Nematodes, e.g. *Trichinella spiralis* and *trichinella pseudospiralis*
Tapeworms	Cestodes, e.g. *Taenia solium* – pork tapeworm *Taenia saginata* – beef tapeworm

Illnesses caused by bacteria

Traveller's diarrhoea

Many people suffer from diarrhoea when they first arrive in a foreign country. It is the most common medical problem for tourists and has been given a variety of descriptive names such as Dehli Belly, the Tandoori Trots, the Kathmandu Quickstep or more simply the Runs.

It is usually caused by *Escherichia coli*, a small rod-shaped bacterium which is present in the intestinal tract of healthy people. Most strains are not pathogenic apart from *E. coli* 0157, which causes serious illness (see p. 54), and a few other strains which cause diarrhoea in babies. Adults are rarely affected except when travelling abroad. Traveller's diarrhoea is usually caused by a strain of *E. coli* which is not found in the traveller's home country but may be widespread in the foreign country. Natives of the country will be unaffected by a similar number of *E. coli* bacteria.

The incubation period is 12–24 hours and the symptoms are abdominal pain, fever, diarrhoea and sometimes vomiting. A healthy adult should recover from traveller's diarrhoea in 2–3 days. No food or a light diet of dry bread, crackers, boiled rice or potatoes with plenty of fluid will settle the symptoms quickly. In severe cases dehydration can be a problem because fluid absorption becomes less efficient when suffering from diarrhoea. The patient should be given a mixture of salt and sugar dissolved in boiled water or a commercial rehydration preparation.

Typhoid fever (also known as enteric fever)

Typhoid fever is caused by *Salmonella typhi*. It is a more severe illness than the food poisoning caused by the majority of species of Salmonella.

Most cases of typhoid fever reported in the UK have been acquired abroad. The incubation period is 7–21 days and the main symptoms are prolonged fever with rose-coloured spots on the body. Severe diarrhoea usually commences in the second or third week of the fever. Typhoid fever is fatal in a small number of cases. After the illness some people become convalescent carriers for months or years.

Causes of the disease

1   Food handlers who are carriers of *Salmonella typhi* and have contaminated food by failing to wash their hands after a visit to the toilet. People who are confirmed carriers of *Salmonella typhi* are not allowed to work in the food industry.

2 Drinking water that has been contaminated by sewage.

3 Shellfish and watercress gathered from sewage-contaminated water. Salads and unwashed fruit.

Paratyphoid fever

Paratyphoid is caused by *Salmonella paratyphi*. It is similar to typhoid but the symptoms are less severe. It is normally acquired by eating food or drinking water which has been contaminated by a human carrier.

Dysentery

Bacillary dysentery is caused by a bacterium called Shigella. It is spread by the faecal–oral route and is a common cause of illness for travellers as well as in the UK (see p. 58).

Vibrio parahaemolyticus food poisoning

Vibrio parahaemolyticus is a comma-shaped bacterium. It is a common contaminant of fish and shellfish in tropical and subtropical waters.

 V. parahaemolyticus is sensitive to heat and is destroyed by thorough cooking. Most cases occur as a result of eating uncooked or undercooked seafood, particularly shellfish.

Incubation period	12–18 hours
Symptoms	Abdominal pain with profuse diarrhoea often with vomiting and fever
Duration	2–5 days

Brucellosis

Brucellosis is acquired by drinking infected unpasteurised cows' or goats' milk.

Incubation period	1–3 weeks
Symptoms	Variable but usually a headache and fever with profuse sweating, loss of appetite, constipation and pain in muscles and joints
Duration	The initial symptoms last approximately 10 days but the fever returns repeatedly for months

Illnesses caused by toxins

Scombrotoxic fish poisoning

Scombrotoxic fish poisoning is usually caused by mackerel, tuna, sardines or pilchards. These fish are rich in the amino acid histidine which is converted to histamine by spoilage bacteria present in the fish. Histamine combines with another substance to form a toxin. Lengthy periods of unrefrigerated storage allow the formation of sufficient toxin in the flesh of the fish to cause symptoms similar to an allergic reaction. The symptoms occur between 15 minutes and three hours after eating the fish and include a burning sensation in the mouth and throat, puffiness around the eyes, swelling of the lips, tongue and gums, urticaria, headache, nausea, vomiting and diarrhoea. They last for 8–12 hours. The toxin is not easily destroyed by heat and canned fish can also cause scombrotoxic fish poisoning.

Paralytic shellfish poisoning

Paralytic shellfish poisoning (PSP) is a serious and sometimes fatal type of food poisoning. It occurs after eating mussels or oysters which have been feeding on a certain type of toxic plankton, resulting in the accumulation of neurotoxins in the flesh of the fish. The toxins can survive cooking.

Symptoms occur between 30 minutes and three hours after eating the fish and include a tingling of the tongue and mouth which spreads to the neck, fingers and toes and occasionally progresses to paralysis. PSP is most likely to occur in exceptionally warm weather.

In some areas, at particular times of year, monitoring of the toxin levels in mussels takes place to establish whether it is safe to harvest them.

Ciguatera poisoning

Ciguatera poisoning can occur following the consumption of warm-water fish such as sea bass, barracuda, grouper and eel which have been feeding on toxin-producing algae. The symptoms include tingling and numbness of the mouth as the fish is eaten. These may progress to respiratory problems and the illness can be fatal.

Illnesses caused by protozoa

Protozoa are single-celled micro-organisms. They live in an aqueous environment, e.g. soil saturated with water, ponds, ditches, rivers and the sea. The majority are harmless but a few are pathogenic to humans.

Giardiasis

Giardiasis is caused by the protozoan *Giardia lamblia*. The illness occurs world-wide but is more common in areas of poor sanitation where water has been contaminated with sewage. Between 4000 and 6000 cases are reported each year in the UK, the majority of which involve tourists returning from abroad.

Incubation period	5–25 days
Symptoms	Profuse watery diarrhoea and abdominal pain

Cryptosporidiosis

The protozoan Cryptosporidium is found in water contaminated with sewage. Cryptosporidiosis is widespread in animals and a common cause of diarrhoea in calves. The infection can be spread in humans by the faecal–oral route or directly from animals to humans. Milk, water and food have also been implicated. Cryptosporidium can survive the pasteurisation process and may survive some water treatment processes. The main symptoms are vomiting, diarrhoea, abdominal pain and fever which last for about 10 days.

Amoebic dysentery

Amoebic dysentery is caused by the protozoan *Entamoeba histolytica*. The disease is spread by the faecal–oral route from infected individuals or from contaminated water or food. The incubation period is usually 3–4 weeks and the main symptoms are abdominal pain and diarrhoea.

This disease is rare in Europe but it is endemic in some tropical countries, particularly in areas of poor sanitation. Between 300 and 1000 cases are reported in the UK each year, the majority of which are travellers returning from abroad.

Illnesses caused by viruses

Hepatitis A and hepatitis E

The strict meaning of hepatitis is inflamed liver. Hepatitis A (also called infective hepatitis) and Hepatitis E are transmitted by food. Hepatitis B can only be transmitted from blood to blood.

Hepatitis A is more likely to be contracted in Middle or Far Eastern countries than in Europe. The incubation period is long (about 2–7 weeks) and the symptoms are fever, nausea, abdominal pain and, later, jaundice. The 'duration' of the illness can be anything from a week to several months and the severity of the symptoms varies considerably.

The virus is spread by the faecal–oral route and so food can be contaminated by a food handler with poor hygiene standards who is a carrier of the virus. Many outbreaks are associated with shellfish collected from sewage-contaminated water.

Polio

The polio virus can be spread via the faecal–oral route. Most people in the UK and other developed countries will have been immunised against this very serious disease as a child. A booster is needed every ten years and all tourists, especially those to countries outside Northern Europe, should ensure that they are up to date with vaccinations.

Illnesses caused by parasitic worms

Worm infections are common in the tropics but occur world-wide, particularly in areas where sewage disposal is inadequate.

Roundworms

Roundworms are the most common worm infection. They are very similar in appearance to the earthworm and grow to a length of 10–30cm. They are usually found in children and are particularly common in Africa and the Far East.

Infection is caused by swallowing the worm's eggs, which may be present in contaminated water or food (often lettuce, fruit and vegetables grown in soil fertilised with human sewage). The eggs grow into worms in the small intestine and then these worms lay eggs which are excreted in the faeces, allowing the cycle of infection to start again. Roundworms may cause mild abdominal symptoms and malnutrition but often the infection is not detected until a worm is passed in the stools. Drug treatment is available and roundworms rarely cause any long-term ill health.

Tapeworms

A tapeworm may grow up to three metres in length in the intestine where it absorbs food, grows and produces eggs which are excreted in the faeces. The tapeworm eggs do not grow into tapeworms in human beings but if they are ingested by cattle or pigs they form cysts in the muscle of the animal. The cysts are usually visible in the meat, giving it a spotted appearance. If the meat is eaten raw or undercooked, the cyst survives and starts to grow into an adult tapeworm in the human intestine.

Humans can act as the intermediary host for the pork tapeworm and if the eggs are ingested, cysts may form in their muscles, eyes or brain. The main symptoms will be fainting and convulsions.

Tapeworm infections can be treated with drugs but a better option is to prevent them by eating only well-cooked meat when travelling in areas of poor sanitation.

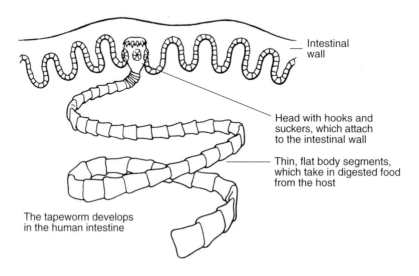

Intestinal wall

Head with hooks and suckers, which attach to the intestinal wall

Thin, flat body segments, which take in digested food from the host

The tapeworm develops in the human intestine

Trichinosis

Trichinosis is caused by a very small worm, *Trichinella spiralis*. The disease is transmitted by pork. The life cycle of the worm is similar to that of tapeworms but the cysts are too small to be seen in the meat.

The symptoms of diarrhoea and abdominal pain start within two days of eating the undercooked pork. One week later, fever, swollen eyes, muscle pains and weakness may appear. Infections can be treated with drugs but they can easily be prevented by only eating well-cooked meat.

Preventive measures

"Boil it, cook it, peel it, shell it or forget it"

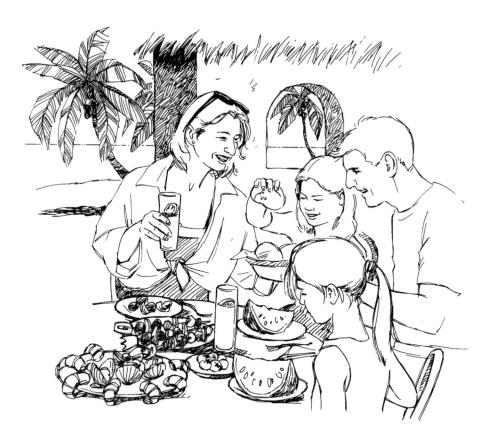

The illnesses contracted abroad as a result of eating and drinking contaminated food are caused by a wide variety of micro-organisms but the ways to avoid these illness are much the same. It is appropriate to use the following advice whichever country is being visited but it is particularly important in areas of poor sanitation.

1   Maintain a high standard of personal hygiene. Avoid eating in restaurants where hygiene standards appear to be poor and hand-washing facilities are inadequate or non-existent. Many of the illnesses described in this chapter are spread by the faecal–oral route.

2   Avoid 'street food' which is often prepared in unhygienic conditions and held at temperatures within the danger zone for long periods of time. It may also have been exposed to flies. However, sizzling hot, thoroughly cooked 'street snacks' are probably safer than lukewarm foods on a hotel buffet table.

3   Drink only boiled water or if this is not possible, drink bottled water. Bottled water is safe in most areas but may not be in areas of poor sanitation. Do not put ice-cubes in drinks unless you are sure they have been made with boiled or good-quality bottled water. Tap water in many areas is contaminated with live micro-organisms. Do not drink milk unless it has been pasteurised. Locally manufactured ice cream should be avoided.

4   Only eat freshly cooked seafood. Avoid eating shellfish as they may have been gathered from sewage-contaminated waters.

5   Avoid eating lettuce and watercress. Salad ingredients with smooth skins such as tomatoes which have been washed in clean water make a better alternative. Always peel fruit and avoid fruit which cannot be peeled, especially those with rough skins which cannot be easily washed such as strawberries and raspberries.

6   Eat only freshly cooked, hot food. Avoid reheated food or food, particularly cooked meats or egg dishes, which have been on display at room temperature for some time. Fried rice is a high-risk food because it is not possible to know the history of the ingredients and flash frying will probably not kill any bacteria present.

PRACTICE EXAMINATION QUESTIONS

1 What are the principal reasons for the increase in the number of cases of food poisoning in the UK?

2 Why are there more outbreaks of food poisoning in the summer months?

3 Are all bacteria harmful? Describe the effects that different types of bacteria have on food.

4 Explain what is meant by:
   (a) binary fission
   (b) bacterial spores
   (c) bacterial toxins
   (d) aerobes and anaerobes.

5 What are the four requirements for bacterial growth? Write a short paragraph about each one.

6 In what ways can food be contaminated whilst being prepared in a kitchen?

7 What is mean by cross-contamination? If you owned a butcher's shop, what advice would you give to your staff to prevent this from occurring?

8 What are the main sources of pathogenic bacteria in the kitchen?

9 Discuss the differences between bacterial food poisoning and bacterial food-borne disease.

10 What precautions would you take when preparing food to ensure that you do not cause Salmonella food poisoning?

11 If you were in charge of preparing sandwiches for a self-service counter, what precautions would you take to minimise the risk of causing staphylococcal food poisoning?

12 Why is the bacterium *Clostridium perfringens* particularly difficult to destroy? What precautions can you take to prevent this type of food poisoning occurring?

13 Why is it particularly important that rice and meat products should not be reheated more than once?

14 Which bacterium causes the majority of cases of diarrhoea in the UK?

15 How does the bacterium *Escherichia coli* cause illness? What are the symptoms and how can you prevent it occurring?

16 Write what you know about the following:
(a) botulism
(b) viral food poisoning
(c) chemical food poisoning.

17 Describe the hand-washing and drying facilities that should be available in a restaurant kitchen.

18 Why is it important to maintain a high standard of personal hygiene when preparing food?

19 Give reasons for the following statements.
(a) Thaw frozen poultry completely before cooking.
(b) Keep food either very hot or very cold.

20 What types of food do not normally cause food poisoning? For each example, explain why this is so.

21 Minced meat dishes are frequently a cause of food poisoning. Give reasons for this.

22 Why are refrigerators important in the prevention of food poisoning? How can you ensure that the temperature of the refrigerator is maintained?

23 Which foods should always be stored in a refrigerator? How would you position the foods you mention and why?

24 Why can food be kept for a longer period of time in a freezer than in a refrigerator? What would you do if your freezer broke down?

25 Describe the cook–chill and cook–freeze methods of food preparation.

26 Describe the different functions of detergents, disinfectants and sanitisers.

27 Describe the different stages in a cleaning and disinfection process.

28 If you were asked to plan a new kitchen, what points regarding the design and layout would you consider important?

29 Why is efficient waste disposal important in a restaurant kitchen and what arrangements would you make to achieve this?

30 What indications would there be of the presence of rats or mice? What action would you take?

31 What are the most common kitchen pests? How can they cause food poisoning?

32 What steps can you take to reduce the risk of an infestation of pests in your premises?

33 What causes food to deteriorate in quality?

34 What is meant by the pH and Aw of food? What effect do they have on bacterial growth?

35 Give details of the main methods of food preservation.

36 What is meant by an HACCP system? What is the advantage of using this approach to food hygiene in a food factory?

37 Describe how you would conduct a hazard analysis in a kitchen providing a cold buffet for 100 people.

38 Outline the requirements of *The Food Safety (General Food Hygiene) Regulations 1995*.

39 What checks will an enforcement officer make during a routine inspection of food premises? What action may he take if conditions are not satisfactory?

40 What advice about food would you give to a student who is planning to spend three months travelling in Asia?

INDEX